Foodie Diary Mexican Recipes - Authentic Mexican CookBook

Adidas Wilson

Published by Financierpro Publishing, 2024.

While every precaution has been taken in the preparation of this book, the publisher assumes no responsibility for errors or omissions, or for damages resulting from the use of the information contained herein.

FOODIE DIARY MEXICAN RECIPES - AUTHENTIC MEXICAN COOKBOOK

First edition. November 4, 2024.

Copyright © 2024 Adidas Wilson.

Written by Adidas Wilson.

To my children,

You are the light that fills my days and the joy that fills my heart. Each of you brings unique magic and boundless love into my life. This work is for you—a reminder of how deeply cherished you are and how much hope and inspiration you give me every day.

May you always follow your dreams, carry kindness in your hearts, and know that you are loved beyond words. You are my greatest accomplishment, my greatest adventure, and my most profound gift. Thank you for being you.

With all my love, always and forever.

"First, we eat tacos. Then, we change the world."

Financierpro, Publishing

P.O. Box 2266

Antioch, Tn. 37011

enterthecrios@gmail.com

www.thefoodiediary.com

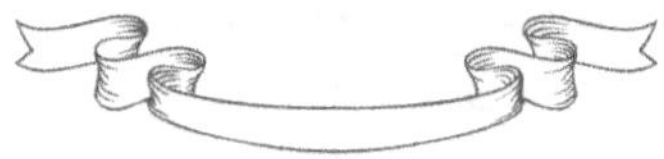

MEXICAN FOOD RECIPES

Discover the rich traditions and bold flavors of Mexican cuisine, from vibrant street eats to celebratory feasts.

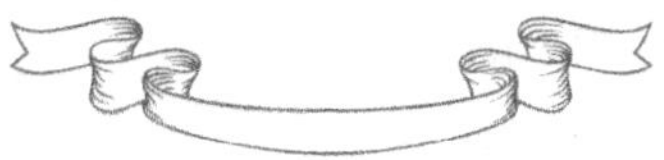

Adidas Wilson

TABLE OF CONTENTS

Introduction

Welcome to the vibrant world of Mexican cuisine! In this cookbook, we're taking you on a flavorful journey through one of the most celebrated culinary traditions in the world. Mexican food is so much more than tacos and burritos—it's a delicious fusion of ancient traditions, local ingredients, and innovative techniques that bring bold flavors to life with every bite. From the bustling street markets of Mexico City to the coastal seafood flavors of Baja California, this cookbook captures the soul of Mexican cooking. Each recipe is crafted to showcase the unique spices, textures, and ingredients that have made Mexican food beloved worldwide. Whether you're a novice cook or a seasoned chef, this collection provides an authentic yet accessible way to experience the diverse range of Mexican cuisine right in your own kitchen. In these pages, you'll find recipes that celebrate classic dishes like enchiladas, tamales, and pozole, alongside regional gems you may not have encountered yet. We'll introduce you to staple ingredients like masa harina, chiles, and fresh herbs that create the foundation of Mexican flavor. You'll also learn about traditional cooking methods, such as nixtamalization, roasting, and charring, that enhance the richness of each dish. Each recipe in this cookbook is inspired by the Mexican culture of family and togetherness, where meals are often shared, savored, and celebrated. So, gather around, and let's embark on this culinary adventure together—because every great meal starts with a love for flavor, a sense of community, and the joy of discovery.

Bienvenidos a la cocina Mexicana! Let's get cooking!

Mexican Food Customs: Rich Traditions and Vibrant Flavors

Mexican food customs are a unique blend of indigenous Mesoamerican traditions and Spanish influences, enriched over centuries to create one of the world's most vibrant and beloved cuisines. Mexican food culture is not just about the flavors and ingredients; it's about community, celebration, and honoring cultural heritage. Mexican food customs vary by region, with each area offering its own local flavors and dishes, but there are certain customs and traditions that unite the Mexican dining experience. Here's a look at some of the key customs, rituals, and foods that make Mexican cuisine so special.

The Importance of Corn, Beans, and Chiles

Corn, beans, and chiles are the foundation of Mexican cuisine and have been essential to Mexican food culture since ancient times. Corn is used in countless forms, from tortillas and tamales to atole (a hot drink) and pozole (a hominy soup). Beans are a staple protein source and are often paired with rice, while chiles add flavor and spice to nearly every Mexican dish. These ingredients are so central to Mexican identity that they appear in traditional stories, mythology, and celebrations.

The Tortilla: A Staple on Every Table

Tortillas, particularly corn tortillas, are a staple at every Mexican meal. Freshly made tortillas are cherished for their flavor and texture, and in many families, making tortillas by hand is a daily tradition. Tortillas accompany nearly every meal and are used in a variety of ways: they're wrapped around fillings to create tacos, rolled and fried to make flautas, layered into enchiladas, and even used as a scoop for salsas and stews. Warm tortillas are served fresh at each meal, often stored in a special basket called a tortillero to keep them warm.

Mealtime Customs: Comida as the Main Meal

In Mexican food culture, comida, or the main meal of the day, is typically eaten in the early afternoon, around 2 to 4 pm. This is a multi-course meal that usually includes soup, rice, a main dish, and dessert. Comida is a time for families to gather, relax, and enjoy a leisurely meal together. Traditionally, la cena (dinner) is a smaller, lighter meal eaten later in the evening, often consisting of a simple soup, salad, or a light snack like tamales or antojitos (snacks).

Sharing Meals and Hospitality

In Mexican culture, food is a way to bring people together. Hospitality and sharing are central values, and food is often prepared for large gatherings to ensure that everyone has plenty to eat. It's common to see family members cooking together, sharing recipes passed down through generations, and spending time around the table. Celebrations, like birthdays, weddings, and holidays, are marked by elaborate meals shared with family and friends. Guests are warmly welcomed, and leaving food on the plate may be seen as impolite, as can be interpreted as a rejection of the host's hospitality.

Street Food and Market Culture

Mexican street food is an integral part of the culinary experience. Markets and street stalls offer a wide array of freshly prepared foods, from tacos and tamales to elote (grilled corn), gorditas, and tortas (Mexican sandwiches). Mercados (markets) are bustling centers of daily life, where people come to buy fresh produce, meat, and spices, and often grab a quick meal at food stalls. Mexican street food is loved for its bold flavors, convenience, and variety, with vendors perfecting their recipes over generations. Eating street food is part of the social fabric and offers an accessible way to sample local specialties.

Celebratory Foods and Traditions

Mexican food customs are rich with traditions surrounding specific holidays and celebrations:

Día de los Muertos (Day of the Dead): This is a time to honor and remember loved ones who have passed away. Families prepare pan de muerto (a sweet, anise-flavored bread) and other favorite foods of the deceased, which are placed on altars as offerings. The foods are often shared among family members to keep the memory of loved ones alive.

Christmas and Las Posadas: During the Christmas season, traditional dishes like tamales, bacalao (salted cod), ponche (a warm fruit punch), and buñuelos (crispy fried pastries) are prepared. Families celebrate Las Posadas with gatherings that include special foods and drinks.

Independence Day: On September 16, Mexicans celebrate their independence with foods that reflect national pride, such as chiles en nogada (stuffed chiles in walnut sauce) and an abundance of red, white, and green dishes that represent the Mexican flag.

Quinceañeras: This is a special celebration marking a girl's 15th birthday. The event includes a lavish meal with traditional foods, like mole, tamales, and a multi-tiered cake. Family and friends gather to celebrate this rite of passage.

Salsas and Condiments

Salsas are indispensable to Mexican cuisine and are served at nearly every meal. Salsa adds flavor, heat, and freshness, and comes in a wide range of varieties—from the spicy, smoky chipotle salsa to the tangy salsa verde made from tomatillos. Hot sauces, pickled chiles, and fresh garnishes like cilantro and onions are also served to complement dishes and allow diners to customize their food to their taste. Many families make their own salsa from scratch, using fresh ingredients and grinding chiles, tomatoes, and herbs in a molcajete (a traditional stone mortar and pestle).

Mexican Drinks: From Aguas Frescas to Tequila

Drinks are an important part of Mexican dining culture. Aguas frescas, refreshing drinks made from fruits, flowers, or grains (like horchata and agua de jamaica), are served with meals to complement the flavors. Mexico is also famous for its spirits, particularly tequila and mezcal, which are made from the agave plant and enjoyed on special occasions. Coffee and hot chocolate are also popular, especially for breakfast or evening gatherings, often made with cinnamon and served with pan dulce (sweet bread).

Respect for Ingredients and Traditional Cooking Methods

Mexican cuisine is deeply rooted in traditional cooking methods that enhance the natural flavors of ingredients. Slow-cooking techniques, like simmering mole or preparing barbacoa, are respected traditions, such as grinding spices by hand and roasting chiles to bring out their smoky essence. Many dishes are prepared with local ingredients specific to a region, celebrating Mexico's rich biodiversity. The use of traditional tools like the comal (a flat griddle) for toasting tortillas and the metate (a stone grinding slab) for grinding corn reflects respect for the cultural and historical significance of food preparation.

The Role of Dessert and Pan Dulce

No Mexican meal is complete without a little something sweet at the end. Pan dulce, or sweet bread, is a staple of Mexican breakfasts and snacks, with varieties like conchas, cuernitos, and empanadas found in every bakery. Desserts like flan, churros, and tres leches cake are also enjoyed after meals or on special occasions. In Mexican culture, enjoying a sweet treat is often part of the social dining experience, and traditional desserts are an important part of holiday celebrations.

Conclusion: Food as a Reflection of Mexican Culture and Community

Mexican food customs are about more than just the food itself; they reflect a deep sense of community, history, and hospitality. Meals are opportunities to gather, celebrate, and connect with family and friends. From simple street tacos to elaborate holiday feasts, Mexican food customs emphasize fresh ingredients, traditional methods, and a love for sharing. By respecting and continuing these food traditions, Mexicans honor their heritage and create meaningful, delicious experiences that bring people together across generations.

Mexican Food Pantry Essentials

Creating authentic Mexican dishes at home begins with stocking a pantry full of traditional ingredients. Mexican cuisine is rich in flavors, colors, and textures, and its pantry essentials reflect this diversity. With a combination of spices, grains, dried chiles, and fresh ingredients, a well-stocked Mexican pantry allows you to prepare a wide array of dishes, from hearty stews to refreshing salsas. Here's a look at the essential ingredients you need to bring the vibrant flavors of Mexico into your kitchen.

Dried Chiles

Dried chiles are a cornerstone of Mexican cooking, used to add depth, heat, and smoky flavor to dishes. Different chiles have unique flavors and heat levels, and they're often rehydrated and blended into sauces, soups, and moles. Here are some common types:

Guajillo Chiles: Mild to medium heat with a fruity, slightly tangy flavor. Guajillos are used in salsa, marinades, and moles.

Ancho Chiles: These are dried poblano peppers with a mild heat and a slightly sweet, raisin-like flavor. Ancho chiles are common in moles and stews.

Pasilla Chiles: Earthy and mildly spicy, pasillas are used in mole, salsas, and soups.

Chipotle Chiles: These are dried and smoked jalapeños, offering a smoky, spicy flavor ideal for salsas, marinades, and sauces.

Masa Harina

Masa harina is a finely ground corn flour made from dried corn that has been treated with lime (nixtamalization), which gives it a unique flavor and texture. Masa harina is essential for making tortillas, tamales, gorditas, and sopes. Simply mix masa harina with water to create a dough, and you're ready to press it into tortillas or shape it into tamales.

Beans

Beans are a staple in Mexican cuisine, providing protein, fiber, and flavor. Common varieties include:

Black Beans (Frijoles Negros): Popular in many Mexican dishes, black beans are used in soups, salads, and as a side dish.

Pinto Beans (Frijoles Pintos): Known for their creamy texture, pinto beans are often used in refried beans, burritos, and stews.

Peruano Beans: Also known as Peruvian beans, these are a bit lighter and softer than pinto beans and are commonly used in central and southern Mexico.

Rice

Rice, especially Mexican rice or Spanish rice, is often served as a side dish or combined with beans. Long-grain white rice is the most used, but brown rice can also work. Mexican rice is typically cooked with tomatoes, onions, garlic, and spices, creating a delicious and slightly tangy flavor.

Corn Tortillas

Corn tortillas are an essential part of Mexican cuisine, used in tacos, enchiladas, chilaquiles, and more. Made from masa harina, they are naturally gluten-free and have a slightly nutty flavor. For an authentic experience, try to find fresh corn tortillas or make them yourself with masa harina. Flour tortillas, though less common in traditional Mexican cooking, are also popular, especially in northern Mexico.

Canned Tomatoes and Tomatillos

Tomatoes and tomatillos are essential for making salsas, sauces, and bases for many Mexican dishes. Canned tomatoes are convenient for making red salsa, rice, and sauces, while tomatillos, which have a tangy flavor, are used to create salsa verde. If fresh tomatillos are not available, canned tomatillos are a great substitute.

Fresh and Dried Herbs

Mexican cuisine uses a variety of fresh and dried herbs to add depth and brightness to dishes:

Cilantro: Fresh cilantro is a key ingredient in salsa, guacamole, and as a garnish for many dishes. Its bright, herbaceous flavor is unmistakable.

Epazote: A strong, earthy herb that's often added to bean dishes to reduce gas and add a distinctive flavor. It's commonly found in Mexican markets and can be used fresh or dried.

Mexican Oregano: Mexican oregano has a slightly citrusy, earthy flavor that differs from Mediterranean oregano. It's used in moles, salsa, and soups.

Spices

Mexican cooking relies on a variety of spices to create complex and robust flavors:

Cumin: Cumin's warm, earthy taste is essential in many Mexican spice blends, salsas, and stews.

Cinnamon (Canela): Mexican cinnamon, or canela, is softer and milder than the cinnamon commonly found in the U.S. It's used in sweet and savory dishes, as well as in drinks like Mexican hot chocolate.

Cloves: Cloves are used in moles, marinades, and stews, adding a warm, slightly sweet flavor.

Allspice: Known as pimienta gorda in Mexico, allspice is used in moles and sauces for its warm, peppery flavor.

Piloncillo

Piloncillo is unrefined cane sugar that comes in cone-shaped blocks. It has a deep, molasses-like flavor and is commonly used in Mexican desserts, drinks, and sauces. To use piloncillo, it's usually grated or melted down with water. Dark brown sugar can be used as a substitute if piloncillo is unavailable.

Chocolate and Cocoa

Mexican chocolate is distinct, often made with cacao, sugar, and cinnamon. It's used to make traditional hot chocolate and is an essential ingredient in mole sauce, where it adds a subtle richness. Cocoa powder can also be used in baking or to create a shortcut mole sauce.

Vinegar and Limes

Mexican food relies on acidic ingredients to balance rich flavors. White vinegar and apple cider vinegar are commonly used in pickling chiles and onions. Fresh limes are an essential ingredient, often squeezed over tacos, soups, and salads to brighten flavors. Lime juice is also essential in marinades and salsa.

Achiote Paste

Achiote paste, made from ground annatto seeds, garlic, spices, and vinegar, is a vibrant red seasoning used in traditional Mexican dishes like cochinita pibil (a slow-roasted pork dish). Achiote has a mild, slightly peppery flavor and adds color to meats, rice, and marinades. It's widely used in Yucatán cuisine.

Stock Cubes or Bouillon

Chicken bouillon or stock cubes are frequently used in Mexican cooking as a flavor enhancer, especially in soups, stews, and rice. Brands like Knorr are popular, and chicken, tomato, or vegetable flavors are common.

Tequila and Mezcal

Though not exactly pantry items, tequila and mezcal are iconic Mexican spirits that are often used in cooking and cocktails. Mezcal has a smoky flavor that adds depth to marinades, sauces, and cocktails, while tequila is commonly used in marinades and dressings and, of course, to make margaritas!

Aguas Frescas Ingredients

Mexican aguas frescas are refreshing drinks made from fruits, flowers, and seeds. To prepare these, it's helpful to have ingredients like:

Hibiscus Flowers (Flor de Jamaica): Dried hibiscus flowers are used to make agua de Jamaica, a tangy, refreshing drink.

Rice: Used to make horchata, a creamy, cinnamon-spiced drink.

Chia Seeds: Often added to agua fresca for texture and nutrition.

Building Your Mexican Pantry

Building a Mexican pantry allows you to explore a variety of dishes and develop a deeper understanding of Mexican flavors. Here's how you can get started:

Start with Staples: Begin by gathering masa harina, beans, rice, dried chiles, and tortillas. These basics will let you prepare many Mexican dishes, from tortillas to tacos to salsas.

Add Flavor Boosters: Stock up on spices like cumin, Mexican oregano, and cinnamon, and don't forget fresh limes, piloncillo, and vinegar to balance flavors.

Explore Sauces and Condiments: Dried chiles, canned tomatoes, and achiote paste will expand your options for creating sauces and marinades.

Expand into Traditional Ingredients: Once you have the essentials, try adding unique ingredients like epazote, hibiscus flowers, and Mexican chocolate to recreate classic dishes and drinks.

Cooking with a Mexican Pantry

With these pantry essentials, you'll have everything you need to make dishes like enchiladas, tamales, mole, and tacos right at home. Mexican cooking is all about layering flavors, balancing spice, and using fresh, vibrant ingredients. Whether you're making salsas, stews, or desserts, a well-stocked Mexican pantry offers endless possibilities to explore and enjoy. Mexican food customs and flavors have stood the test of time, and building a Mexican pantry is a great way to experience and honor these culinary traditions. With a combination of basic staples, spices, fresh herbs, and specialized ingredients, your kitchen can be ready for any Mexican dish, bringing the authentic taste of Mexico to your table.

Mexican Herbs and Spices

Mexican cuisine is known for its bold and complex flavors, many of which come from a variety of herbs and spices that are unique to this cuisine. The right blend of herbs and spices brings life to Mexican dishes, adding warmth, depth, and brightness. Here's a guide to some of the most essential herbs and spices used in Mexican cooking, each of which plays a key role in creating the vibrant flavors of Mexican dishes.

Mexican Oregano (Orégano Mexicano)

Mexican oregano differs from the Mediterranean oregano commonly found in North America and Europe. It has a more robust, citrusy, and earthy flavor with a slightly peppery undertone. Mexican oregano is used in a variety of dishes, from salsas and soups to stews and beans. It pairs particularly well with chiles and tomatoes and is a key ingredient in moles, pozole, and tacos.

Usage Tip: Use Mexican oregano in dried form and crush it between your fingers before adding it to dishes to release its full flavor.

Epazote

Epazote is an herb with a strong, earthy, and slightly medicinal flavor that is unique to Mexican cuisine. It's commonly used in dishes that include beans, as it is believed to reduce gas and aid digestion. Epazote's distinctive taste also complements dishes like quesadillas, tamales, and certain Mexican sauces.

Usage Tip: Fresh epazote is preferred, but it can be difficult to find outside of Mexico. Dried epazote works as a substitute but use it sparingly as its flavor is intense.

Cilantro (Coriandrum sativum)

Cilantro, also known as coriander leaves, is one of the most used herbs in Mexican cooking. Known for its bright, citrusy flavor, cilantro is used fresh as a garnish for tacos, soups, and salsa and in dishes like guacamole and ceviche. It adds freshness and a subtle bitterness that balances spicy and savory flavors.

Usage Tip: Add fresh cilantro at the end of cooking to preserve its flavor and aroma. Use both leaves and stems for an extra boost of flavor.

Cumin (Comino)

Cumin is a warm, earthy spice that adds depth and smokiness to Mexican dishes. It's a key component in many spice blends and is used to season meats, beans, stews, and rice. Cumin is often toasted before grinding, which enhances its flavor and adds a rich aroma to dishes.

Usage Tip: Use ground cumin sparingly, as its flavor can be overpowering. For an authentic taste, toast whole cumin seeds and grind them yourself.

Cinnamon (Canela)

Mexican cinnamon, or canela, is different from the cinnamon commonly used in the United States. It comes from a softer bark and has a milder, sweeter, and more delicate flavor. Canela is used in both sweet and savory Mexican dishes, such as mole, churros, and café de olla (Mexican spiced coffee).

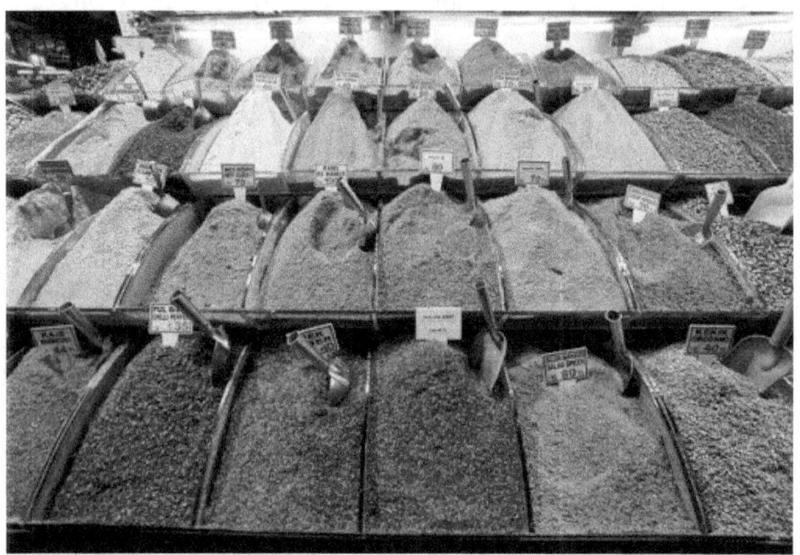

USAGE TIP: USE MEXICAN cinnamon sticks rather than ground cinnamon for a more authentic flavor and add them to simmering dishes to release their sweetness gradually.

Allspice (Pimienta Gorda)

Allspice, known as pimienta gorda or "fat pepper" in Mexico, has a flavor reminiscent of cloves, cinnamon, and nutmeg. It's used in moles, marinades, and stews, and its warm, peppery flavor is ideal for creating depth in sauces and broths. Allspice is often found in Mexican spice blends and is also used to season meats.

Usage Tip: Whole allspice berries are best for simmering in broths and sauces. For a stronger flavor, grind them fresh before adding them to dishes.

Cloves (Clavo de Olor)

Cloves add a warm, sweet spice to Mexican dishes, particularly in marinades, moles, and sauces. Their strong flavor can dominate a dish, so they are used sparingly. Cloves are also popular in Mexican desserts, where they complement cinnamon and allspice.

Usage Tip: Use whole cloves in simmering dishes and sauces, removing them before serving, or grind them fresh for marinades and spice blends.

Anise Seed (Anís)

Anise seed has a sweet, licorice-like flavor that is used in both sweet and savory Mexican dishes. It's commonly used in bread, such as pan de muerto, as well as in certain traditional candies and beverages. Anise adds a subtle, sweet note that pairs well with cinnamon and cloves.

Usage Tip: Add a small amount of anise seed to dishes, as its flavor is strong. Toasting it lightly before use can bring out its sweetness.

Bay Leaves (Hojas de Laurel)

Bay leaves add an earthy, slightly floral flavor to soups, stews, and sauces. In Mexican cuisine, they are often used in broths, beans, and moles. They're typically simmered in the liquid and removed before serving.

Usage Tip: Use dried bay leaves for a mellow, slow-release flavor. Add them early in the cooking process to allow their flavor to develop fully.

Achiote (Annatto)

Achiote, also known as annatto, is a spice made from the seeds of the achiote tree. It has a mild, earthy, and slightly peppery flavor and is commonly used as a natural coloring agent. Achiote paste, made by grinding annatto seeds with spices, is used in dishes like cochinita pibil and gives them a vibrant red-orange hue.

Usage Tip: Dissolve achiote paste in citrus juice or vinegar to create a marinade or use it to add color and flavor to rice and sauces.

Coriander Seeds (Semillas de Cilantro)

Coriander seeds come from the same plant as cilantro but have a completely different flavor profile—earthy, citrusy, and slightly nutty. They are often toasted and ground to season meats, beans, and sauces. Coriander seeds add a subtle depth to dishes and complement cumin in spice blends.

Usage Tip: Toast whole coriander seeds before grinding to bring out their aromatic oils and enhance their flavor.

Chiles (Fresh and Dried)

Chiles are not only a source of heat but also add flavor, smokiness, and complexity to Mexican dishes. Here are some commonly used chiles:

Jalapeño: A fresh, moderately spicy chile used in salsas, toppings, and marinades.

Serrano: Smaller and spicier than jalapeños, serranos are commonly used in salsas and sauces.

Poblano: A mild chile often roasted and used in dishes like chiles rellenos or in sauces after drying (ancho chile).

Guajillo, Ancho, Pasilla, and Chipotle: Dried chiles used to add depth and smokiness to sauces, moles, and marinades.

Usage Tip: Each chile offers a unique flavor. Rehydrate dried chiles in hot water before blending them into sauces, and experiment with different varieties to create complex flavors.

Garlic (Ajo)

Garlic is a fundamental ingredient in Mexican cooking, used to add depth and aroma to nearly every savory dish. It's often combined with onions, tomatoes, and chiles to create a flavor base for sauces, stews, and marinades.

Usage Tip: Sauté garlic in oil to release its flavor, or roast it for a milder, sweeter taste.

Thyme (Tomillo)

Thyme is used in Mexican cooking to add an earthy, slightly minty flavor to dishes, especially in broths, stews, and marinades. It's often paired with bay leaves and oregano to create a savory base for complex dishes like birria and certain moles.

Usage Tip: Use dried thyme for a subtle flavor, adding it early in cooking so it has time to infuse the dish.

Marjoram (Mejorana)

Marjoram is like oregano but has a sweeter, milder flavor. It's often used alongside thyme and bay leaves in Mexican spice blends and is particularly common in dishes like pozole, caldo de res, and menudo. Marjoram adds a delicate floral note that enhances the flavors of meat and broths.

Usage Tip: Use dried marjoram sparingly in broths and stews to add complexity without overpowering other flavors.

Crafting Authentic Mexican Flavors

Mexican herbs and spices are fundamental to the cuisine, each contributing unique flavors that add warmth, richness, and depth. Whether you're simmering a pot of pozole, blending a homemade mole, or garnishing a bowl of tacos, these herbs and spices allow you to create authentic Mexican flavors in your kitchen.

Start by building a spice collection that includes Mexican oregano, cumin, cinnamon, and dried chiles. Then, experiment with more unique herbs like epazote, achiote, and allspice to expand your flavor palette. Mexican cooking is all about balancing flavors—heat, acidity, sweetness, and earthiness—and these herbs and spices are the keys to achieving that balance.

By stocking your pantry with these essentials and learning how to use them, you can create traditional Mexican dishes that honor the country's culinary heritage, bringing the vibrant, complex flavors of Mexico to your table.

Essential Mexican Dry Ingredients

Mexican cuisine is known for its rich flavors and textures, many of which come from dry ingredients that have been used for centuries. From the aromatic dried chiles that bring smokiness and heat to dishes, to corn-based products like masa harina that serve as the foundation for tortillas, these pantry staples are key to creating authentic Mexican dishes. Here's a look at the essential Mexican dry ingredients you should have in your pantry to capture the traditional flavors of Mexico.

Masa Harina

Masa harina is a finely ground corn flour made from dried corn that has been nixtamalized (treated with lime). It's the essential base for making tortillas, tamales, gorditas, and sopes. Masa harina is simply mixed with water to form a dough, creating the signature texture and taste that's unique to Mexican cuisine.

Usage Tip: Choose a high-quality masa harina specifically labeled for tortillas or tamales. For the best results, follow package instructions for the right water-to-flour ratio.

Dried Chiles

Dried chiles are a staple of Mexican cooking, bringing depth, heat, and complexity to sauces, soups, and stews. Different chiles offer unique flavors and levels of spiciness, and they're often rehydrated and blended to create classic Mexican sauces.

Guajillo Chiles: Mild to medium heat with a fruity, slightly tangy flavor. Commonly used in salsa, moles, and marinades.

Ancho Chiles: Mild, with a rich, slightly sweet taste. Ancho chiles are dried poblano peppers and are used in moles, adobos, and stews.

Pasilla Chiles: Earthy and mild, pasillas are popular in moles and sauces, especially in combination with other chiles.

Chipotle Chiles: Smoked and dried jalapeños with a medium heat and smoky flavor. They're ideal for adding depth to salsa, marinades, and sauces.

Usage Tip: To bring out their full flavor, lightly toast dried chiles in a pan before rehydrating them in warm water. Then, blend them into sauces or salsa.

Beans

Beans are a staple protein source in Mexican cuisine and are commonly used in soups, stews, and as a side dish. They add texture, flavor, and nutrition to meals.

Black Beans: Earthy and slightly sweet, black beans are used in soups, burritos, tacos, and as a side dish.

Pinto Beans: Creamy and mild, pinto beans are popular in re-fried beans and stews.

Peruano (Peruvian) Beans: Also known as canary beans, they're lighter in color and have a buttery texture, often used in central and southern Mexican dishes.

Usage Tip: Soak dried beans overnight for quicker cooking and to reduce the gas-producing compounds. Adding epazote to beans while cooking is a traditional method believed to aid digestion.

Cornmeal and Corn Grits

While masa harina is made from nixtamalized corn, regular cornmeal and corn grits are also used in Mexican cooking. Cornmeal is used for making cornbread, tamal-style cornbreads, or even crusts. Coarse corn grits are sometimes added to soups for extra texture.

Usage Tip: Cornmeal can be used to coat fish or chicken for a Mexican-style crust, adding a subtle sweetness and crunch.

Rice

Rice is a staple side dish in Mexican cuisine and is often paired with beans or served with main dishes. Mexican rice, or Spanish rice, is typically cooked with tomatoes, onions, and garlic to create a flavorful accompaniment to many meals.

Usage Tip: For the best Mexican rice, sauté the rice in oil before adding the liquid, which helps prevent it from becoming mushy and adds a slightly nutty flavor.

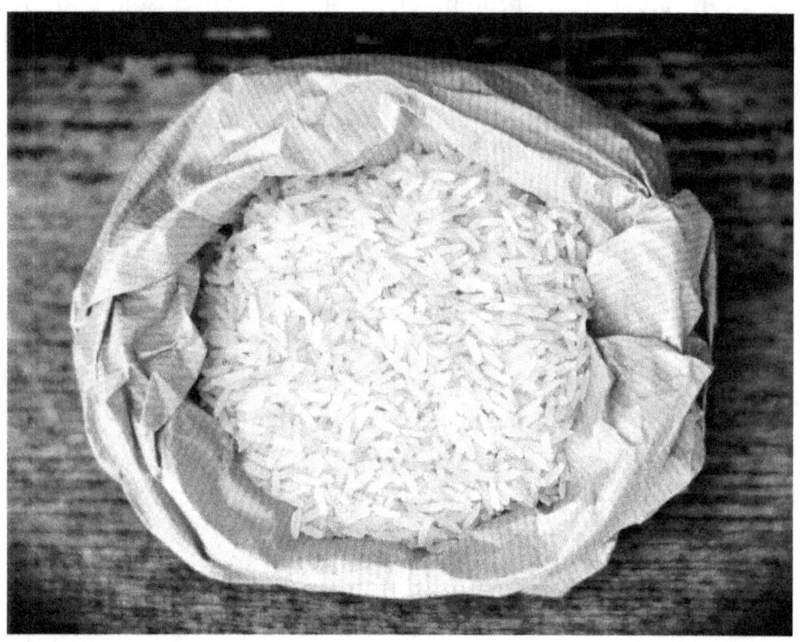

PILONCILLO

Piloncillo is unrefined cane sugar that comes in hard, cone-shaped blocks. It has a deep molasses-like flavor and is used in both sweet and savory dishes, including sauces, desserts, and drinks like atole and café de olla.

Usage Tip: Grate or chop piloncillo before using it, as it can be quite hard. To dissolve it, simmer with water to create syrup for use in recipes.

Dried Herbs

Mexican cuisine relies on several key dried herbs for distinctive flavor:

Mexican Oregano: Unlike Mediterranean oregano, Mexican oregano has a citrusy, earthy flavor. It's used in moles, soups, and stews.

Epazote: Known for its unique, slightly medicinal flavor, epazote is used primarily in bean dishes. It's available to dry if you can't find fresh.

Thyme: Often used in combination with bay leaves and oregano in broths and stews, thyme adds an earthy warmth to dishes.

Usage Tip: Rub dried herbs between your fingers before adding them to dishes to release their oils and enhance their flavor.

Achiote (Annatto) Powder or Paste

Achiote, made from annatto seeds, has a mild, peppery flavor and a vibrant red color. Achiote paste, which is often combined with vinegar, garlic, and spices, is used in dishes like cochinita pibil and gives foods a beautiful reddish-orange color.

Usage Tip: Dissolve achiote paste in citrus juice or vinegar to make a marinade for meats or add to rice and stews for color and flavor.

Spices

Mexican cuisine uses a variety of spices to add warmth and depth to dishes. Some of the most essential spices include:

Cumin: Earthy and slightly smoky, cumin is a core spice in Mexican food, used in everything from taco seasoning to bean dishes.

Cinnamon (Canela): Mexican cinnamon, or canela, has a milder, sweeter flavor than the common cassia cinnamon. It's used in both savory and sweet dishes.

Cloves: Used in small amounts, cloves add a warm spice to moles, adobos, and marinades.

Allspice: Known as pimienta gorda, allspice adds a unique warmth and is often used in moles and marinades.

Usage Tip: Toast whole spices in a dry pan before grinding to enhance their flavor in dishes.

Dried Chiles de Árbol

Chiles de árbol are small, slender red chiles with a fiery heat. They are often used to add spice to salads, sauce, and infused oils.

They're also ground into powder for sprinkling on dishes for extra heat.

Usage Tip: Use chiles de árbol sparingly as they are very spicy. To soften their heat, remove the seeds before cooking with them.

Corn Husks

Corn husks are used primarily for making tamales, as they serve as the wrapper for the masa and fillings. They add a subtle corn flavor and aroma to tamales during steaming.

Usage Tip: Soak corn husks in warm water for about 30 minutes before using them for tamales. This makes them pliable and easy to work with.

Stock Cubes or Bouillon

Chicken, beef, or tomato bouillon cubes are commonly used in Mexican cuisine to enhance the flavors of rice, stews, and soups. Brands like Knorr are popular in Mexico, and they add a rich umami taste to dishes.

Usage Tip: Use bouillon cubes sparingly, as they are often high in salt. Adjust additional seasonings accordingly.

Dried Hibiscus Flowers (Flor de Jamaica)

Dried hibiscus flowers are used to make agua de jamaica, a tart, refreshing drink with a beautiful ruby color. Hibiscus is also used in sauces, desserts, and marinades, as it adds a tangy flavor like cranberries.

Usage Tip: To make agua de jamaica, steep the dried flowers in hot water, then sweeten to taste. Strain before serving.

Tamarind Pods or Paste

Tamarind adds a tangy, slightly sweet flavor to Mexican candies, drinks, and sauces. Tamarind paste is made from tamarind pods and is often mixed with sugar for balance. It's a popular ingredient in agua fresca and certain marinades.

Usage Tip: If using tamarind pods, soak them in warm water and strain out the seeds and pulp to create a smooth paste.

Hibiscus Powder and Dried Herbs

Herbs like epazote, Mexican oregano, and thyme add depth to stews, beans, and soups. Dried herbs offer convenience and concentrated flavor, making them pantry staples for many Mexican households.

Usage Tip: When using dried herbs in beans or soups, add them early in the cooking process to allow their flavors to infuse the dish.

Building Your Mexican Pantry

To create authentic Mexican flavors, stock your pantry with these essential dry ingredients. Start with staples like masa harina, dried chiles, beans, and rice, then add spices, dried herbs, and flavor enhancers like bouillon and piloncillo. These dry ingredients provide a solid foundation for Mexican dishes, from tacos and tamales to refreshing beverages and bold sauces. With these dry ingredients in your pantry, you'll have everything you need to explore the rich, complex flavors of Mexican cuisine and bring traditional dishes to life in your own kitchen.

The Role of Dairy in Mexican Cuisine

Dairy products in Mexican cuisine are used to enhance flavors, provide creamy textures, and balance the heat of spicy dishes. Cheeses and creams are commonly used as toppings, fillings, or integral components of recipes. Dairy not only adds richness but also contributes to the nutritional value of meals, offering protein and calcium.

Mexican Cheeses (Quesos)

Mexican cheeses are distinct in flavor and texture, often made from cow's milk, goat's milk, or a combination of both. They range from fresh and mild to aged and sharp, each serving a specific purpose in cooking.

Queso Fresco

Description: Queso fresco is fresh, crumbly cheese with a mild, slightly salty flavor.

Uses: Commonly crumbled over dishes like tacos, enchiladas, and salads. It doesn't melt well but adds a creamy texture when heated.

Cotija Cheese

Description: Named after the town of Cotija in Michoacán, this aged cheese has a strong, salty flavor and a crumbly texture like Parmesan.

Uses: Sprinkled over elote (grilled corn), beans, soups, and salads. It's often referred to as the "Parmesan of Mexico."

Oaxaca Cheese

Description: A semi-soft, stringy cheese like mozzarella, Oaxaca cheese is known for its melting properties and mild, buttery flavor.

Uses: Ideal for quesadillas, empanadas, and chiles rellenos due to its excellent melting ability.

Queso Panela

Description: A fresh, white cheese with a smooth texture and mild taste. Panela doesn't melt but softens when heated.

Uses: Often sliced and grilled or fried, used in sandwiches, or served with fruit and salads.

Chihuahua Cheese

Description: Originating from the state of Chihuahua, this cheese is pale yellow with a mild, buttery flavor and excellent melting properties.

Uses: Perfect for queso fundido (melted cheese dip), casseroles, and stuffed dishes.

Queso Añejo

Description: An aged version of queso fresco, queso añejo is firm, salty, and sharp in flavor.

Uses: Grated over dishes as a finishing touch, like how one might use Romano or Parmesan cheese.

Requesón

Description: Like ricotta cheese, requesón is a soft, grainy cheese made from the whey left after making other cheeses.

Uses: Used in fillings for empanadas, enchiladas, and pastries.

Mexican Creams and Dairy Toppings

Crema Mexicana

Description: A rich, thick cream like crème fraîche, but slightly sweeter and less tangy than sour cream.

Uses: Drizzled over tacos, enchiladas, soups, and desserts to add a creamy texture and mellow spicy flavors.

Crema Agria

Description: The Mexican version of sour cream, crema agria is tangier and less thick than crema Mexicana.

Uses: Used similarly to Crema Mexicana but provides a tangier taste that complements rich and spicy dishes.

Milk and Other Dairy Products

Leche Condensada and Leche Evaporada

Description: Sweetened condensed milk (leche condensada) and evaporated milk (leche evaporada) are concentrated milk products used in desserts and beverages.

Uses: Essential in making tres leches cake, flan, and certain types of atole (a traditional hot corn-based beverage).

Cajeta

Description: A sweet confection made from goat's milk caramelized with sugar, like dulce de leche but with a distinct flavor.

Uses: Drizzled over desserts like churros, crepes, ice cream, and used as a filling in pastries.

Rompope

Description: A traditional Mexican eggnog-like beverage made with milk, sugar, egg yolks, spices, and often rum or brandy.

Uses: Served as a festive drink during holidays and used as a flavoring in desserts.

Dairy in Traditional Mexican Dishes

Enchiladas Suizas: Corn tortillas filled with chicken and covered with a creamy tomatillo sauce and melted cheese.

Chiles Rellenos: Poblano peppers stuffed with cheese (often Oaxaca or Chihuahua) and sometimes meat, then battered and fried.

Quesadillas: Tortillas filled with melting cheeses like Oaxaca or Chihuahua and grilled until the cheese is gooey.

Elote (Mexican Street Corn): Grilled corn on the cob slathered with crema Mexicana or mayonnaise, cotija cheese, chili powder, and lime juice.

Sopes and Gorditas: Thick corn masa cakes topped with beans, meats, lettuce, crema, and crumbled queso fresco or cotija.

Flan: A creamy custard dessert made with eggs, milk, and caramelized sugar, sometimes incorporating condensed or evaporated milk for richness.

Tres Leches Cake: A sponge cake soaked in a mixture of three milks—evaporated milk, condensed milk, and heavy cream—topped with whipped cream.

Regional Variations

Different regions in Mexico have their own specialties when it comes to dairy products:

Jalisco: Known for birria topped with fresh cheeses and served with crema.

Oaxaca: Famous for Oaxaca cheese and traditional dishes like tlayudas (large, toasted tortillas topped with beans, cheese, and meats).

Chiapas: Produces a variety of fresh cheeses used in local cooking.

Michoacán: Renowned for cotija cheese and dishes that highlight its sharp flavor.

Dairy products are integral to Mexican cuisine, adding richness, texture, and balance to a wide array of dishes. From the crumbly cotija cheese enhancing the flavor of elote to the creamy sweetness of cajeta drizzled over desserts, these ingredients showcase the diversity and depth of Mexican culinary traditions. Understanding and utilizing these dairy products can elevate your cooking and provide an authentic taste of Mexico's rich food heritage.

Frequently Asked Questions

Q: Can I substitute Mexican cheeses with more readily available cheeses in recipes?

Yes, while Mexican cheeses provide authentic flavor and texture, you can substitute them if they're not available. For example, feta can replace cotija, mozzarella can substitute for Oaxaca cheese, and ricotta can stand in for requesón.

Q: Where can I find Mexican dairy products?

Many Mexican dairy products are available at Latin American grocery stores or the international aisle of larger supermarkets. Some specialty cheese shops may also carry them. Additionally, online retailers offer a selection of Mexican cheeses and creams.

Q: What is the difference between crema Mexicana and sour cream?

Crema Mexicana is richer and less tangy than sour cream, with a thinner consistency. Sour cream (crema agria) is tangier and thicker. While they can often be used interchangeably, crema Mexicana is preferred for its ability to mellow spicy flavors without overpowering the dish.

Q: Are there dairy-free alternatives in Mexican cuisine?

While traditional Mexican cuisine relies on dairy in many dishes, you can find or create dairy-free versions by substituting cheeses with plant-based alternatives and using dairy-free creams made from nuts or soy. Many authentic dishes, like salsas, guacamole, and certain bean dishes, are naturally dairy-free.

Q: What is cajeta, and how is it different from dulce de leche?

Cajeta is a type of caramel made from goat's milk, giving it a unique flavor profile compared to dulce de leche, which is made from cow's milk. Cajeta has a slightly tangier taste and is a specialty of the state of Guanajuato in Mexico. By incorporating these Mexican dairy products into your cooking, you can explore new flavors and textures that bring authenticity and richness to your dishes. Whether you're topping tacos with crumbled queso fresco or enjoying a slice of tres leches cake, these ingredients are sure to enhance your culinary experience.

Essential Mexican Tools and Equipment

Mexican cuisine is rich, diverse, and full of unique flavors that are often achieved through traditional cooking techniques. From grinding spices to preparing tortillas and moles, having the right tools and equipment can make all the difference in recreating authentic Mexican dishes at home. Here's a guide to some of the most essential tools used in Mexican cooking, each of which plays a role in bringing traditional flavors and textures to life.

Molcajete and Tejolote (Mexican Mortar and Pestle)

The molcajete, a traditional Mexican mortar, is typically made of volcanic stone, which gives it a rough texture ideal for grinding ingredients. The tejolote, or pestle, is used to grind spices, chiles, garlic, herbs, and other ingredients to make salsa, guacamole, and marinades.

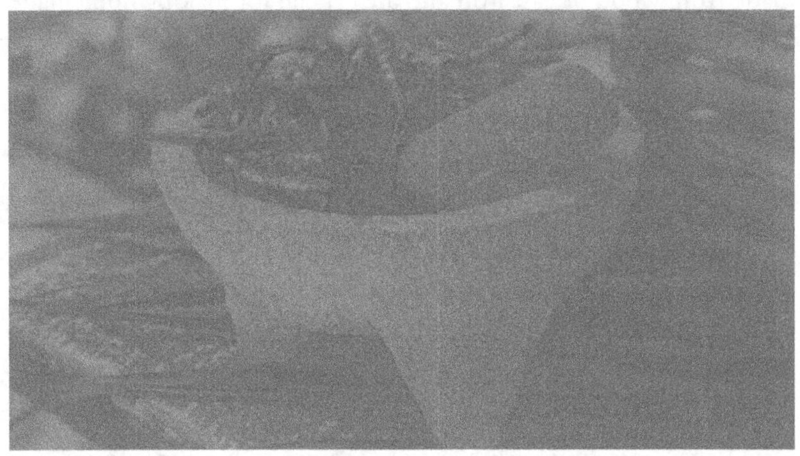

USAGE: MOLCAJETES ARE perfect for grinding ingredients to create thick, textured sauces with a rustic feel. They are also known to enhance flavor by releasing essential oils through grinding.

Tips: Before using a new molcajete, season it by grinding rice or coarse salt to remove stone particles.

Comal

The comal is a flat, round griddle traditionally made of cast iron or clay, used in Mexican cooking to toast tortillas, roast chiles, and cook ingredients like tomatoes and garlic. It's an essential tool for preparing tortillas, quesadillas, and toasting ingredients for salsa and moles.

Usage: Heat tortillas, toast spices, and char vegetables on the comal to enhance their flavor.

Tips: Preheat the comal over medium heat to prevent sticking. If using a clay comal, avoid high heat and sudden temperature changes, as they can cause it to crack.

Tortilla Press (Prensa para Tortillas)

A tortilla press is a device used to flatten balls of masa (corn dough) into thin, round tortillas. Traditional tortilla presses are made from wood or cast iron and are crucial for making homemade corn tortillas.

Usage: Place a ball of masa between two pieces of plastic or parchment paper in the press, then press down to flatten.

Tips: For the best results, line the press with plastic wrap or parchment paper to prevent the dough from sticking.

Metate y Mano (Stone Grinding Slab and Roller)

The metate is a traditional Mexican tool used for grinding corn, cacao, and spices. It consists of a large, flat stone slab and a hand-held cylindrical roller. The metate is ideal for creating the coarse textures of masa, moles, and chocolate.

Usage: Grinding with a metate requires a back-and-forth motion. It's labor-intensive but gives ingredients a unique texture.

Tips: Like the molcajete, the metate should be seasoned before first use by grinding rice or salt to smooth the surface.

Tamalera (Steamer Pot)

A tamalera is a large, often cylindrical, steamer pot specifically designed for steaming tamales. It has a rack inside to keep the tamales above the boiling water and allows for even cooking.

Usage: Fill the pot with water below the steaming rack, arrange tamales vertically, and steam with the lid on.

Tips: Line the rack with corn husks or a damp cloth to keep tamales moist and prevent them from sticking.

Cazuela (Earthenware Pot)

The cazuela is a clay pot often used for slow-cooking dishes like moles, beans, stews, and adobos. Clay pots retain heat well and add an earthy flavor to dishes, making them ideal for traditional Mexican recipes.

Usage: Use the cazuela for simmering and slow cooking, which enhances flavors in complex dishes.

Tips: Soak a new cazuela in water for several hours before first use to prevent cracking.

Olla de Barro (Clay Bean Pot)

An olla de barro is a clay pot traditionally used for cooking beans. The porous nature of clay allows beans to cook evenly and imparts a subtle earthy flavor that's difficult to replicate with other cookware.

Usage: Soak beans overnight, then simmer them in the olla de barro with water and seasonings for tender, flavorful beans.

Tips: Avoid sudden temperature changes, as they can crack the pot. Clean it by rinsing with warm water, as soap can seep into the clay.

Churro Maker

A churro maker, or churro press, is a tool used to pipe churro dough into the traditional long, star-shaped sticks before frying. While not essential, it's a handy tool for making homemade churros.

Usage: Fill the churro maker with dough, then squeeze to pipe it directly into hot oil for frying.

Tips: Work quickly and carefully when frying churros to ensure even cooking.

Molino (Hand Mill)

A molino, or hand mill, is used for grinding grains like corn to make masa for tortillas, tamales, and other corn-based dishes. Although many people now use electric mills, traditional molinos are still used in Mexican households.

Usage: Place the dried corn or grains in the molino and crank the handle to grind it into masa or flour.

Tips: Keep the mill clean and adjust the settings as needed for coarse or fine grinds.

Molinillo (Mexican Wooden Whisk)

A molinillo is a traditional Mexican whisk used to froth hot chocolate and other beverages. This wooden whisk is rolled between the palms to create a foamy top on drinks, adding a unique texture.

Usage: Place the molinillo in a pot of hot chocolate, roll it between your palms, and froth until foamy.

Tips: Use a molinillo with traditional Mexican hot chocolate tablets, which are often flavored with cinnamon for an authentic experience.

Tortillero (Tortilla Warmer)

A tortillero is a small basket, often lined with cloth, used to keep tortillas warm and soft. It's commonly made of woven palm leaves, plastic, or ceramic and is essential for serving fresh tortillas at the table.

Usage: Line the tortillero with a cloth or napkin, place warm tortillas inside, and cover to retain heat.

Tips: For the best results, wrap the tortillas in a damp cloth inside the tortillero to keep them moist.

Canasta de Tamales (Tamale Basket)

A canasta de tamales is a basket used for transporting and keeping tamales warm. It's traditionally lined with cloth or leaves and is often used by vendors and families to carry tamales for gatherings or celebrations.

Usage: Place the tamales inside the lined basket, cover, and keep warm for serving.

Tips: Lining the basket with banana leaves or corn husks adds aroma and keeps tamales warm.

Espátula de Madera (Wooden Spatula)

A wooden spatula is a simple yet essential tool for stirring and flipping food on the comal or in a cazuela. Wooden utensils are gentle on clay cookware and help to avoid scratching nonstick surfaces.

Usage: Use the espátula to stir sauces, flip tortillas, and scrape the bottom of clay pots without damaging them.

Tips: Wash wooden utensils by hand and avoid soaking them for long periods to extend their lifespan.

Mantequera (Butter Keeper or Cheese Mold)

A mantequera is a small mold used for making fresh cheese, like queso fresco or requesón. It shapes the cheese while allowing excess liquid to drain, helping create a firm, textured cheese.

Usage: Line the mold with cheesecloth, fill with curds, press gently, and let it drain.

Tips: If you don't have a mantequera, you can use a small bowl lined with cheesecloth to shape and drain fresh cheeses.

Regional Variations in Cooking Tools

While these tools are widely used throughout Mexico, some regions have specialized equipment unique to their local cuisine:

Yucatán: Often uses a grill called a parrilla to cook foods like cochinita pibil, which is traditionally cooked underground.

Oaxaca: Known for its traditional stone mills and clay comales, used to prepare dishes like tlayudas and mole.

Central Mexico: Uses cazuelas extensively to cook moles and stews due to their ability to retain and distribute heat evenly.

Traditional Mexican cooking relies on a variety of specialized tools and equipment, each designed to bring out the authentic flavors and textures of the cuisine. From grinding spices in a molcajete to pressing tortillas and steaming tamales, these tools add an element of artistry and authenticity to the cooking process. Incorporating these tools into your kitchen will allow you to experience the unique techniques and flavors of Mexican cuisine right at home.

Frequently Asked Questions

Q: Can I use a regular frying pan instead of a comal?

Yes, a cast-iron skillet can be used as a substitute for a comal. However, a comal's flat, unglazed surface provides the ideal texture for toasting tortillas and roasting chiles.

Q: Do I need a tortilla press to make tortillas?

While a tortilla press makes it easier to achieve thin, even tortillas, you can also use a heavy dish or rolling pin. Place the dough between plastic wrap for a clean press.

Q: How do I clean a molcajete?

Rinse with warm water and scrub with a brush. Avoid using soap, as it can seep into the stone and affect future flavors.

Q: Is it essential to use clay cookware for Mexican dishes?

Not essential, but clay pots enhance flavors, especially for beans and stews. If you don't have clay cookware, use a slow cooker or heavy pot.

By incorporating these traditional tools into your kitchen, you can enjoy a more authentic and immersive experience with Mexican cooking, bringing the country's rich culinary heritage to life in your own home.

Traditional Mexican Breakfast

Mexican breakfasts are flavorful, hearty, and diverse, drawing from fresh ingredients and bold spices that make mornings a true delight. From savory egg dishes to filling corn-based meals and sweet treats, a traditional Mexican breakfast offers a variety of dishes that satisfy all tastes. Here's a look at some iconic Mexican breakfast recipes you can try at home, complete with step-by-step instructions for each.

Chilaquiles

Chilaquiles are a classic Mexican breakfast that consists of tortilla chips topped with red or green salsa, cheese, crema, and other garnishes. Often served with fried eggs or shredded chicken, chilaquiles are hearty, flavorful, and comforting.

Ingredients

8-10 corn tortillas, cut into triangles

Vegetable oil, for frying

1 cup salsa verde or salsa roja (homemade or store-bought)

1/2 cup crumbled queso fresco or shredded cheese

1/4 cup Mexican crema or sour cream

1/4 cup chopped onion

Fresh cilantro, for garnish

2 eggs, fried (optional)
Instructions

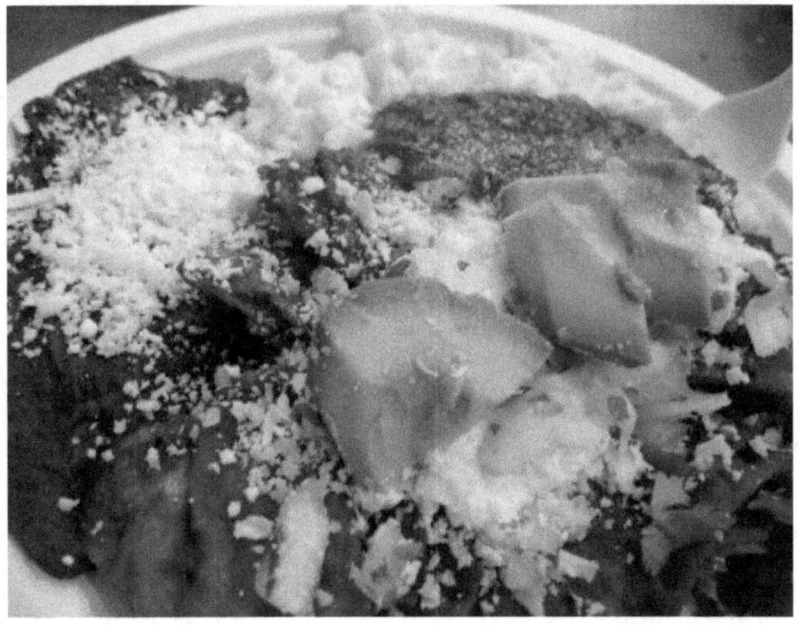

FRY THE TORTILLAS: Heat vegetable oil in a skillet over medium-high heat. Fry the tortilla triangles in batches until they're crispy and golden. Drain on paper towels and set aside.

Simmer in Salsa: In a large skillet, heat the salsa over medium heat until it simmers. Add the fried tortillas, stirring gently to coat them with the salsa. Cook for 2-3 minutes until the tortillas soften slightly but are still crispy.

Serve and Garnish: Divide the chilaquiles onto plates. Top with crumbled queso fresco, a drizzle of crema, chopped onions, and fresh cilantro. Serve with a fried egg on top for added protein.

Huevos Rancheros

Huevos rancheros, or "ranch-style eggs," is a popular breakfast dish featuring fried eggs served on tortillas with a layer of refried beans and topped with salsa. It's a simple yet flavorful dish that highlights traditional Mexican ingredients.

Ingredients

4 corn tortillas

1 cup refried beans (homemade or canned)

4 eggs

1 cup salsa (homemade or store-bought)

1/4 cup crumbled queso fresco

Fresh cilantro, for garnish

Salt and pepper, to taste

Vegetable oil, for frying

Instructions

Prepare the Tortillas: In a skillet over medium-high heat, warm each tortilla for 1-2 minutes on each side. Set them aside and keep warm.

Cook the Eggs: In the same skillet, add a bit of oil and fry the eggs until the whites are set but the yolks are still runny. Season with salt and pepper.

Assemble the Huevos Rancheros: Spread a layer of refried beans on each tortilla. Top with a fried egg, a spoonful of salsa, and a sprinkle of queso fresco. Garnish with fresh cilantro and serve immediately.

Molletes

Molletes are open-faced breakfast sandwiches made with crusty bread topped with refried beans, melted cheese, and pico de gallo. They're deliciously savory and quick to prepare, perfect for a filling breakfast.

Ingredients

4 bolillo rolls, split in half (or use crusty baguette slices)

1 cup of refried beans

1 cup shredded cheese (like Oaxaca, Monterey Jack, or Chihuahua cheese)

Pico de gallo, for topping (tomato, onion, cilantro, and lime juice)

Salt and pepper, to taste

Instructions

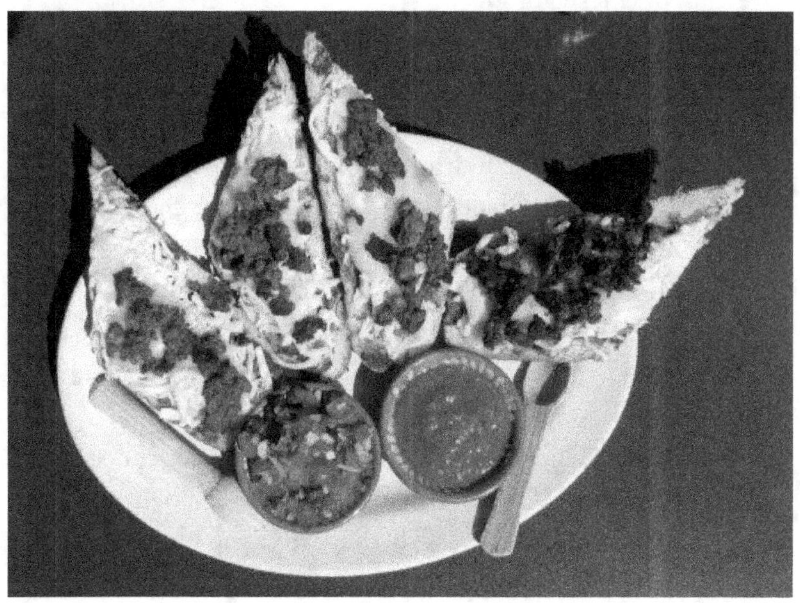

PREPARE THE BREAD: Preheat your oven to 350°F (175°C). Place the bolillo halves on a baking sheet, cut side up.

Assemble the Molletes: Spread a layer of refried beans on each bread half. Sprinkle shredded cheese on top.

Bake: Bake for about 5-7 minutes, or until the cheese is melted and bubbly.

Top and Serve: Remove from the oven, top each mollete with pico de gallo, and season with salt and pepper to taste. Serve warm.

Tamales

Tamales are traditional Mexican breakfast items made from masa (corn dough) filled with meats, cheese, or chiles, and steamed in corn husks. They're perfect for a hearty breakfast and can be made in large batches for convenience.

Ingredients

2 cups of masa harina

2 cups of chicken broth

1/2 cup lard or vegetable shortening

1 tsp baking powder

1/2 tsp salt

Corn husks, soaked in warm water for 1 hour

Filling of choice (shredded chicken with salsa, cheese, or rajas (sliced poblano peppers))

Instructions

Prepare the Masa Dough: In a large bowl, mix the masa harina, baking powder, and salt. Add the lard and chicken broth gradually, mixing until the dough is smooth and spreadable.

Assemble the Tamales: Take a soaked corn husk and spread a small amount of masa dough in the center. Add a spoonful of your chosen filling. Fold the sides of the husk over the filling, then fold the bottom up to close.

Steam the Tamales: Arrange the tamales upright in a steamer pot. Cover and steam for about 1 to 1 1/2 hours, or until the masa is firm and pulls away from the husk easily.

Serve: Allow the tamales to cool slightly before unwrapping and serving.

Atole and Champurrado

Atole is a warm, thickened drink made from masa harina, milk, and cinnamon, and champurrado is a chocolate version of atole. Both are comforting, rich, and perfect for chilly mornings, often served with tamales.

Ingredients for Atole

4 cups milk

1/2 cup masa harina

1/4 cup piloncillo or brown sugar

1 cinnamon stick

1 tsp vanilla extract

Ingredients for Champurrado (Chocolate Atole)

4 cups milk

1/2 cup masa harina

1/4 cup piloncillo or brown sugar

1 cinnamon stick

2 oz Mexican chocolate, chopped

Instructions

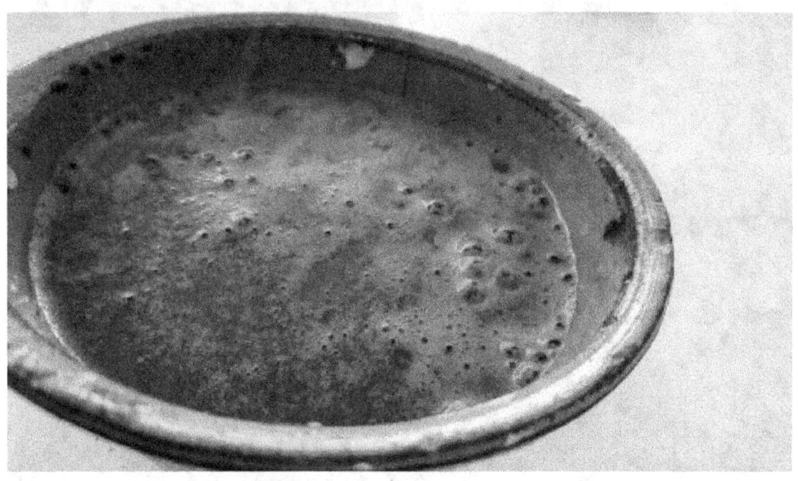

HEAT THE MILK: IN A saucepan, heat the milk and cinnamon stick over medium heat until warm.

Mix Masa Harina: In a small bowl, whisk the masa harina with a bit of water until smooth. Add this to the milk, stirring constantly to avoid lumps.

Add Sweetener and Flavorings: Add piloncillo (or brown sugar) and vanilla extract. For champurrado, add the Mexican chocolate. Stir until fully dissolved and the drink thickens slightly.

Serve Warm: Remove the cinnamon stick and pour the atole or champurrado into mugs. Enjoy it with tamales or pan dulce (sweet bread).

Pan Dulce (Sweet Bread)

Mexican sweet bread, or pan dulce, is a beloved breakfast treat. From conchas (shell-shaped bread) to empanadas and orejas, pan dulce is usually served with coffee or hot chocolate. You can find pan dulce in Mexican bakeries, but here's a recipe for the classic conchas.

Ingredients

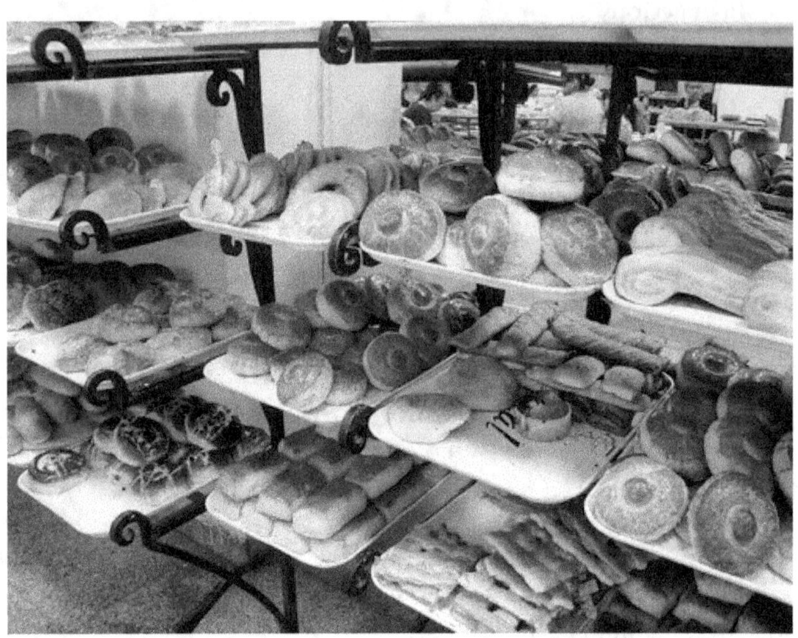

1 CUP WARM MILK

     2 1/4 tsp active dry yeast

     1/3 cup of sugar

     1/2 tsp salt

     2 large eggs

     4 cups of all-purpose flour

     1/2 cup of butter, softened

Topping Ingredients
1/2 cup of butter
1/2 cup powdered sugar
1/2 cup all-purpose flour
Food coloring (optional)

Instructions

Make the Dough: In a bowl, combine warm milk, yeast, and sugar. Let it sit until foamy, about 5 minutes. Add salt, eggs, and flour, mixing until the dough forms. Knead for 5-7 minutes, then add butter and continue kneading until smooth. Let rise until doubled.

Prepare the Topping: Mix butter, powdered sugar, and flour to create the topping. Divide and add food coloring if desired.

Shape and top the Conchas: Divide the dough into 12 balls and place on a baking sheet. Flatten slightly, then top each with a round of the topping. Use a knife to score shell-like patterns.

Bake: Bake at 350°F (175°C) for 15-20 minutes or until golden.

Traditional Mexican breakfasts are vibrant, filling, and rich in flavors. From savory options like chilaquiles and huevos rancheros to comforting drinks like atole and sweet treats like pan dulce, each dish offers a glimpse into Mexico's diverse culinary heritage. These breakfast recipes provide a hearty start to the day and showcase the warmth and complexity that Mexican cuisine brings to the table. Whether you're craving something savory, sweet, or warm and comforting, these recipes will help you create a delicious Mexican breakfast at home.

Antojitos: Mexican Street Food

Antojitos, meaning "little cravings" in Spanish, are Mexican street foods that capture the heart of the country's vibrant and flavorful cuisine. These delicious treats are often enjoyed as snacks, appetizers, or even light meals. Made from corn masa and topped with various ingredients, antojitos are the perfect example of Mexican ingenuity and creativity, showcasing diverse flavors, textures, and traditional ingredients.

Here's a look at some of the most beloved antojitos you'll find across Mexico, along with a few recipes to bring the taste of Mexican street food into your own kitchen.

Tacos

Tacos are perhaps the most well-known Mexican street food, with endless varieties to choose from. They start with a soft corn or flour tortilla and are filled with meats like carnitas (pork), carne asada (grilled beef), or al pastor (spit-grilled pork with pineapple), as well as veggies, salsas, and garnishes.

How to Make Basic Street Tacos

Ingredients:

Corn tortillas

1 lb carne asada, al pastor, or carnitas

Chopped onions, cilantro, and radishes

Lime wedges

Salsa of choice

Instructions:

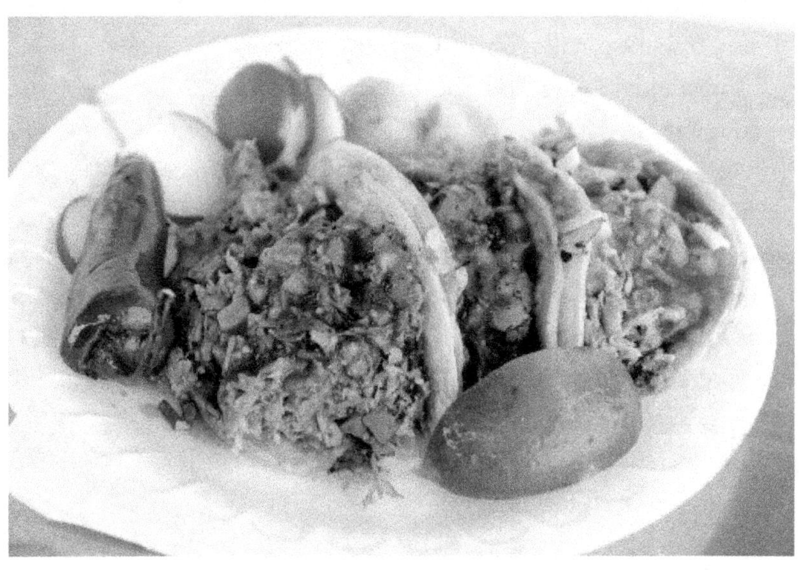

HEAT TORTILLAS ON A skillet until warm and pliable.

Fill each tortilla with a small amount of meat, top with chopped onions, cilantro, and radishes.

Serve with lime wedges and salsa.

Tostadas

Tostadas are crispy, flat corn tortillas topped with layers of beans, meat, lettuce, cheese, and salsa. The base is usually fried or baked until crisp, making it a deliciously crunchy vehicle for flavorful toppings.

How to Make Tostadas

Ingredients:

Corn tortillas

Refried beans

Shredded chicken or beef

Shredded lettuce

Crumbled queso fresco or shredded cheese

Salsa, sour cream, and sliced avocado for topping

Instructions:

Fry or bake tortillas until crisp and golden.

Spread a layer of refried beans on each tostada, followed by the shredded meat.

Add lettuce, cheese, and any toppings you like, such as salsa, sour cream, and avocado.

Sopes

Sopes are thick, round corn masa cakes with raised edges to hold savory toppings. These masa boats are filled with beans, meat, lettuce, crema, and cheese, making them a satisfying snack or meal.

How to Make Sopes

Ingredients:

2 cups of masa harina

1 1/4 cups warm water

Refried beans, cooked meat, shredded lettuce, and cheese for topping

Mexican crema

Instructions:

In a bowl, combine masa harina and water until the dough forms. Divide into small balls and flatten slightly.

Cook on a hot skillet for 2-3 minutes on each side until lightly browned.

While warm, pinch the edges to create a small rim.

Top with refried beans, meat, lettuce, cheese, and a drizzle of crema.

Gorditas

Gorditas, meaning "little fatties," are thick, stuffed masa pockets that are split open and filled with savory ingredients. Popular fillings include cheese, chicharrón (pork cracklings), or rajas (poblano strips).

How to Make Gorditas

Ingredients:

2 cups of masa harina
1 1/4 cups warm water
Fillings like cheese, refried beans, or chicharrón
Instructions:

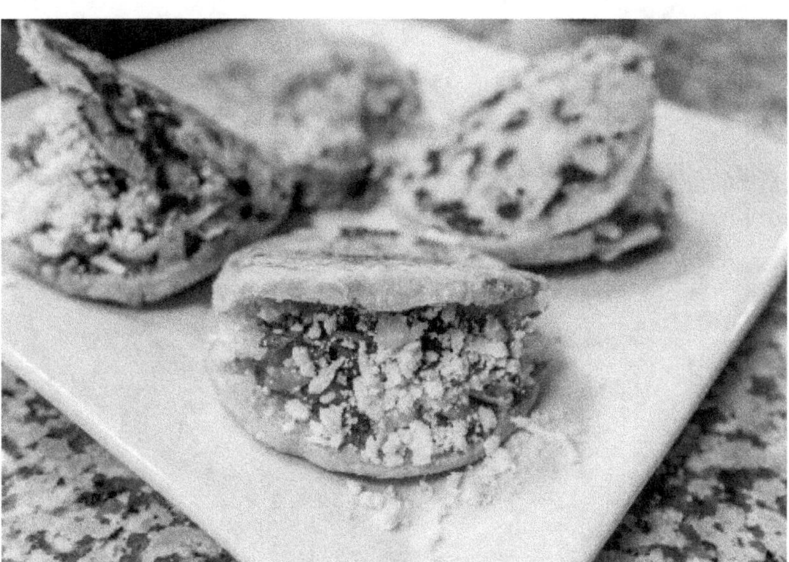

MIX MASA HARINA AND water to form a dough. Divide into balls and flatten to a 1/2-inch thickness.

Cook on a skillet until browned on both sides, about 4-5 minutes per side.

Carefully slice open each gordita and stuff with desired fillings.

Tlacoyos

Tlacoyos are oval-shaped masa cakes that are stuffed before being cooked. Traditionally filled with ingredients like refried beans, fava beans, or cheese, tlacoyos are then topped with nopales (cactus), salsa, and cheese.

How to Make Tlacoyos
Ingredients:
2 cups of masa harina

1 1/4 cups warm water
Refried beans or cheese for filling
Nopales, salsa, and queso fresco for topping
Instructions:

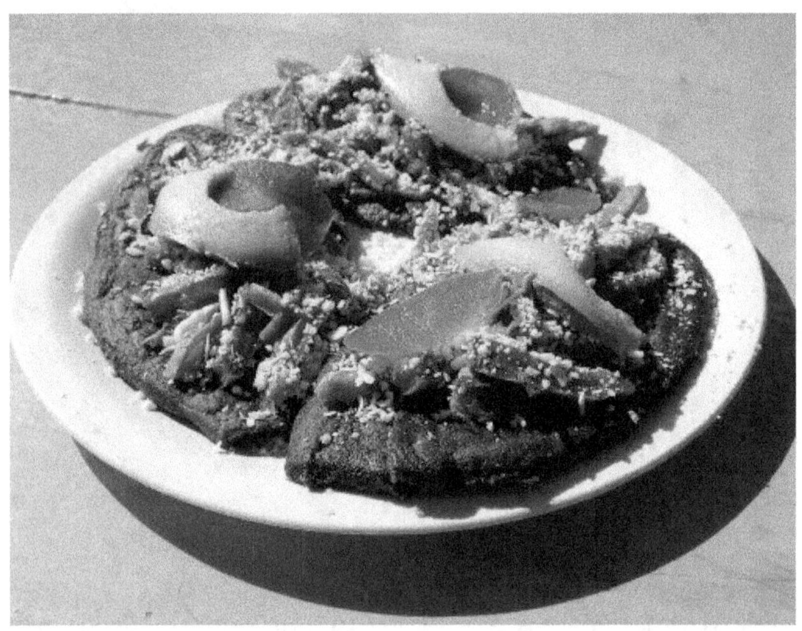

MIX MASA HARINA AND water to form a dough. Divide into balls and flatten into an oval shape.

Place a small amount of filling in the center, fold the masa over, and seal the edges.

Cook on a hot skillet until golden brown on each side.

Top with nopales, salsa, and queso fresco.

Elote and Esquites

Elote (grilled corn on the cob) and esquites (corn kernels served in a cup) are popular street foods that showcase the natural sweetness of corn. Both are topped with mayonnaise, cheese, chili powder, and lime juice for a savory, tangy flavor.

How to Make Elote and Esquites

Ingredients:

Corn on the cob (for elote) or corn kernels (for esquites)

Mayonnaise

Crumbled cotija cheese

Chili powder

Lime wedges

Instructions:

For elote, grill the corn until charred. For esquites, sauté corn kernels in a skillet until tender.

Top with mayonnaise, cotija cheese, chili powder, and a squeeze of lime.

Quesadillas

In Mexico, quesadillas can be made with or without cheese, filled with a variety of ingredients like mushrooms, flor de calabaza (squash blossoms), or huitlacoche (corn fungus). They're typically made with corn tortillas and cooked on a comal (griddle) until the filling is warm and melty.

How to Make Mexican Quesadillas

Ingredients:

Corn tortillas

Cheese, mushrooms, or other fillings of choice

Salsa for dipping

Instructions:

Place filling in a corn tortilla, fold in half, and press gently.

Cook on a comal over medium heat until the tortilla is crispy and the filling is warm.

Serve with salsa.

Tamales

Tamales are corn masa dough stuffed with meats, cheese, or vegetables, wrapped in corn husks, and steamed. They often enjoyed during holidays and celebrations but are also popular street food.

How to Make Basic Tamales

Ingredients:

2 cups of masa harina

2 cups of chicken broth

1/2 cup lard or vegetable shortening

Fillings (like shredded chicken with salsa)

Corn husks, soaked in warm water

Instructions:

Combine masa harina, lard, and chicken broth until smooth.

Spread masa on a soaked corn husk, add filling, and fold the husk around the masa.

Steam tamales for about 1-1.5 hours or until firm.

Empanadas

Empanadas are stuffed pastry turnovers that can be savory or sweet. Fillings range from picadillo (ground beef with spices) to cheese and sweet fruit.

How to Make Empanadas

Ingredients:

Pre-made or homemade empanada dough

Fillings like cheese, meat, or fruit

Egg wash for brushing

Instructions:

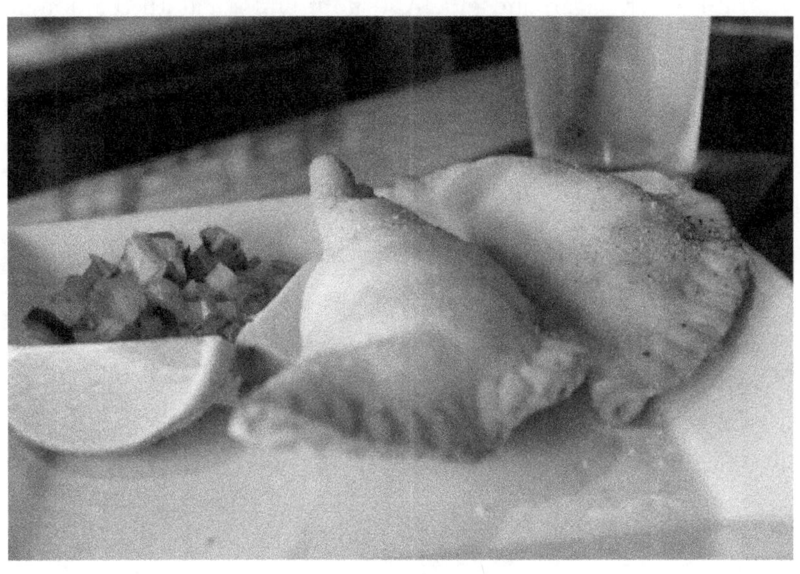

ROLL OUT DOUGH AND cut into circles.

Place filling in the center, fold in half, and seal the edges.

Brush with egg wash and bake at 350°F until golden.

Churros

Churros are long, fried dough pastries coated in sugar and sometimes cinnamon. Crispy on the outside and soft on the inside, they are served with chocolate or caramel sauce for dipping.

How to Make Churros

Ingredients:

1 cup of water

2 tbsp sugar

1/2 tsp salt

1 cup flour

Oil for frying

Sugar and cinnamon for coating

Instructions:

Boil water, sugar, and salt. Add flour and stir until the dough forms.

Pipe the dough into hot oil using a star-shaped nozzle. Fry until golden.

Roll in sugar and cinnamon and serve with chocolate sauce.

Pambazos

Pambazos are soft, dipped sandwiches filled with potatoes and chorizo, then fried until golden. They're soaked in red guajillo chile sauce, which gives them their distinctive color and flavor.

How to Make Pambazos

Ingredients:

Guajillo chile sauce

Soft bread rolls

Potato and chorizo filling

Lettuce, crema, and cheese for topping

Instructions:

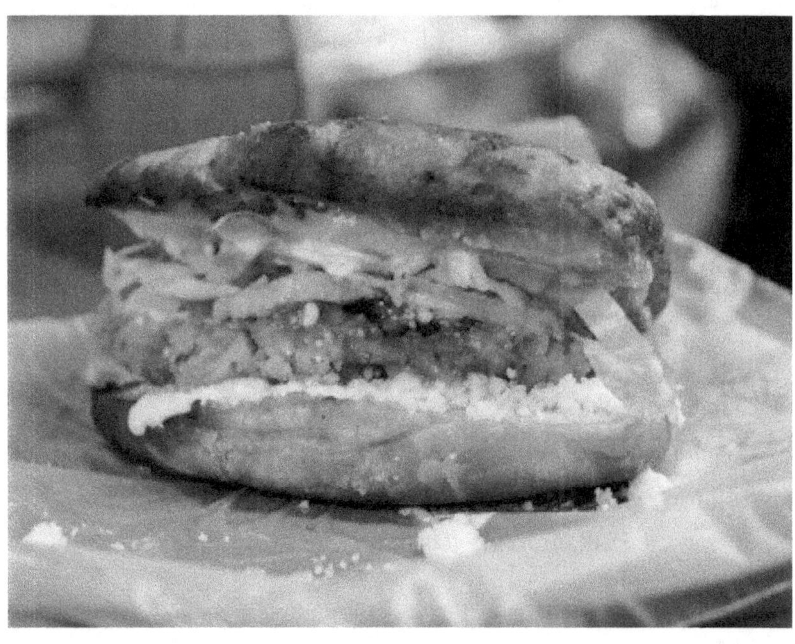

DIP EACH ROLL IN GUAJILLO sauce and fry in a skillet until golden.

Split the bread, add the potato-chorizo filling, and top with lettuce, crema, and cheese.

Antojitos are more than just snacks; they're a celebration of Mexican street food culture, offering endless combinations of flavors, textures, and ingredients. Each antojito tells a story and brings people together, whether at family gatherings, street food stalls, or community events. With these recipes, you can bring the joy of Mexican street food into your own kitchen, experimenting with different toppings, fillings, and flavors to create your perfect antojito experience.

Popular Mexican Drinks

Mexican drinks are as vibrant and diverse as the country's cuisine. From refreshing fruit-based aguas frescas to traditional fermented beverages and iconic spirits, Mexican drinks showcase the creativity and deep cultural heritage of the country. Whether you're looking for something light and refreshing or bold and warming, Mexican beverages offer something for every occasion. Here's a guide to some of Mexico's most popular drinks, complete with descriptions and recipes for a few you can make at home.

Aguas Frescas

Aguas frescas are refreshing, lightly sweetened drinks made from water, fruit, flowers, or grains. They're especially popular during the summer and are a staple in Mexican markets and street stalls. Common flavors include agua de jamaica (hibiscus), agua de horchata (rice and cinnamon), and agua de tamarindo (tamarind).

How to Make Agua de Jamaica (Hibiscus Water)

Ingredients:

1 cup dried hibiscus flowers

4 cups of water

1/2 cup sugar (or to taste)

Ice and lime wedges, for serving

Instructions:

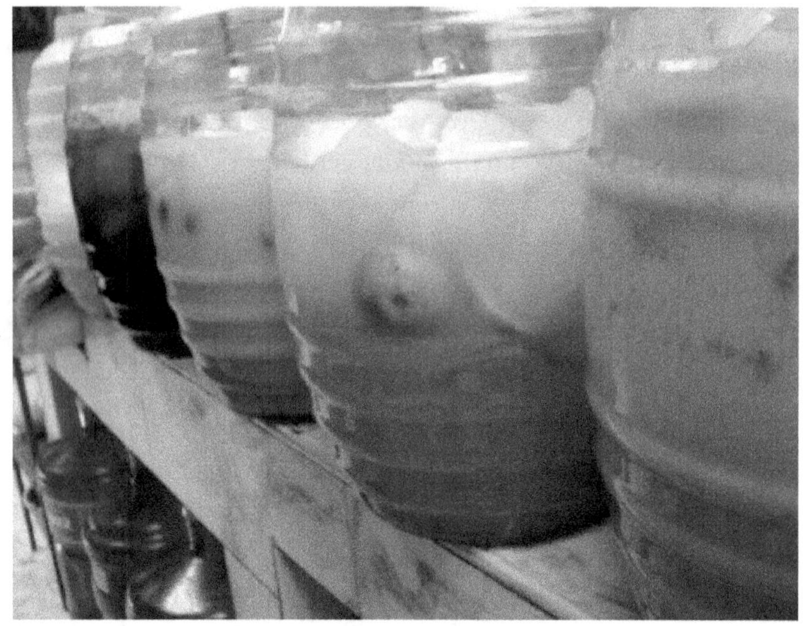

BOIL 4 CUPS OF WATER, add hibiscus flowers, and simmer for 10 minutes.

Strain and discard the flowers, then add sugar to the hot liquid and stir to dissolve.

Allow it to cool, then pour over ice and serve with lime wedges.

Horchata

Horchata is a creamy, rice-based drink flavored with cinnamon and sweetened with sugar. It's a deliciously cool and comforting drink, often enjoyed with spicy dishes to help balance the heat.

How to Make Horchata

Ingredients:

1 cup rice, rinsed

4 cups of water

1 cinnamon stick

1/2 cup of sugar

1 cup milk

1 tsp vanilla extract

Instructions:

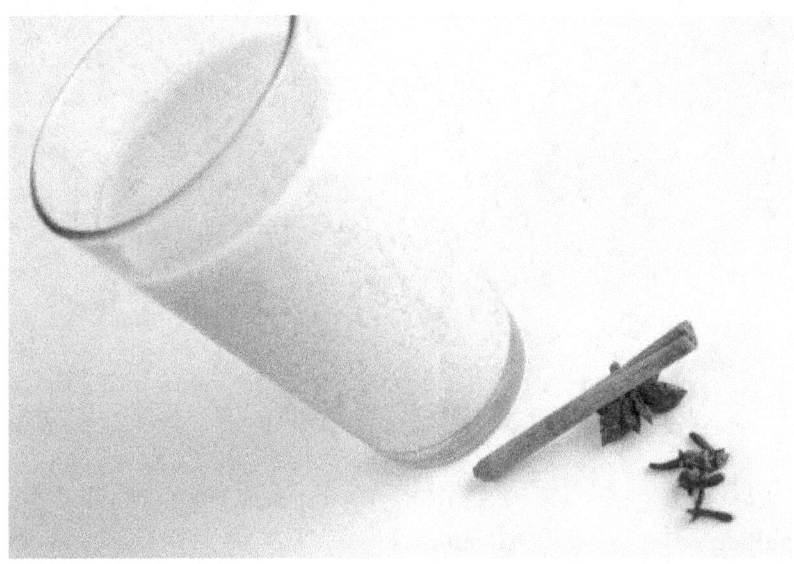

SOAK THE RICE AND CINNAMON stick in water overnight. Blend the soaked rice mixture, then strain through a fine sieve. Add sugar, milk, and vanilla extract. Stir well and serve over ice.

Agua de Tamarindo

Agua de tamarindo is a tangy, slightly sweet drink made from tamarind pods. The tamarind's natural sourness gives this drink a refreshing and unique flavor, perfect for hot days.

How to Make Agua de Tamarindo

Ingredients:

10-12 tamarind pods

4 cups of water

1/2 cup sugar (or to taste)

Instructions:

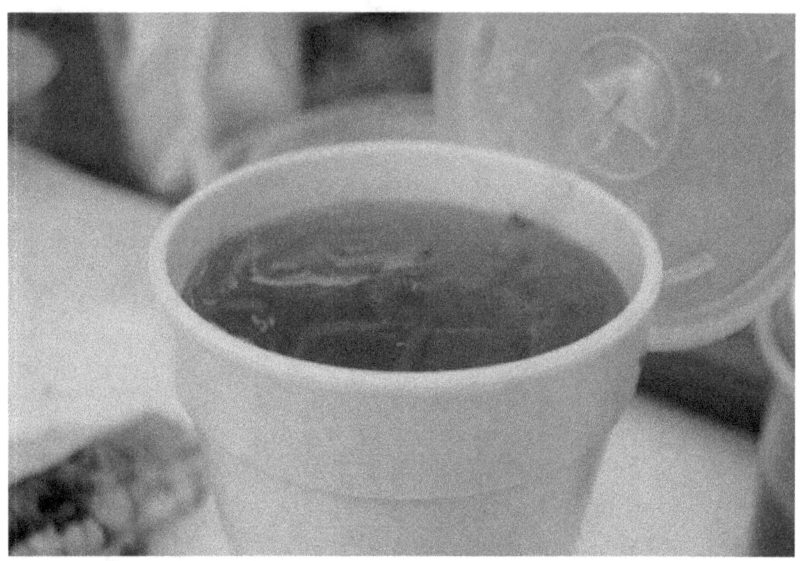

REMOVE THE SHELLS FROM the tamarind pods and boil the pulp in water for about 10 minutes.

Mash the pulp to extract the juice, strain out the solids, and add sugar.

Stir until the sugar dissolves, let cool, and serve over ice.

Mexican Hot Chocolate

Mexican hot chocolate is a rich, frothy drink made with cacao, cinnamon, and sometimes a hint of chili. It's traditionally frothed using a wooden whisk called a molinillo, creating a creamy texture that makes it ideal for cold mornings or evenings.

How to Make Mexican Hot Chocolate

Ingredients:

4 cups of milk

1-disc Mexican chocolate (like Abuelita or Ibarra)

1 cinnamon stick

A pinch of chili powder (optional)

Instructions:

Heat milk in a saucepan with the cinnamon stick until hot but not boiling.

Add the chocolate disc and stir until it melted. Use a molinillo or whisk to create a frothy top.

Pour into mugs, add a pinch of chili powder if desired, and enjoy!

Tejuino

Tejuino is a fermented corn drink popular in western Mexico, particularly in Jalisco. It's made from masa (corn dough) mixed with piloncillo (unrefined cane sugar) and is often served with a scoop of lime sorbet or a squeeze of lime juice.

How Tejuino is Made

To make tejuino, masa is dissolved in water and boiled with piloncillo until it thickens. The mixture is then allowed to ferment slightly, which gives it a unique tangy flavor. It's typically served over ice with lime for a refreshing, slightly sour taste.

Pulque

Pulque is an ancient Mexican alcoholic drink made from the fermented sap of the agave plant. Known as the "drink of the gods," pulque has a long history in indigenous Mexican culture. It has a thick, milky appearance and a slightly tangy flavor, and it's often flavored with fruit or spices.

Pulque is hard to find outside Mexico due to its short shelf life, but it remains popular in pulquerías (pulque bars) throughout the country. Today, you can find many flavored versions, such as pulque de piña (pineapple) and pulque de avena (oatmeal).

Mezcal

Mezcal is a smoky, distilled spirit made from the heart of the agave plant. While tequila is a type of mezcal made specifically from blue agave, mezcal can be made from a variety of agave plants, giving it a wider range of flavors. Mezcal is traditionally enjoyed straight, often with a slice of orange and a sprinkle of chili powder or salt.

How to Enjoy Mezcal: Sip mezcal slowly to appreciate its smoky complexity. Pair it with fresh fruit or spicy snacks for a true Mexican experience.

Tequila

Tequila is one of Mexico's most famous exports and is a type of mezcal made exclusively from blue agave in designated regions of Mexico. Tequila can be enjoyed in a variety of ways: as a shot with lime and salt, in a margarita, or sipped straight.

Types of Tequila:

Blanco (Silver): Unaged, fresh, and full of agave flavor.

Reposado (Rested): Aged for 2-12 months, with a smooth, balanced flavor.

Añejo (Aged): Aged for 1-3 years, with deep, complex flavors.

Michelada

Michelada is a refreshing beer-based cocktail that combines light Mexican beer with lime juice, tomato juice, hot sauce, and spices. It's served over ice in a salt-rimmed glass and is a popular choice on hot days or as a hangover cure.

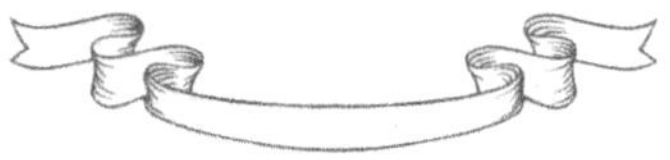

HOW TO MAKE A MICHELADA

Ingredients:

1 bottle of light Mexican beer (like Modelo or Corona)

Juice of 1 lime

1/4 cup tomato juice or Clamato

Hot sauce, Worcestershire sauce, and soy sauce to taste

Salt and chili powder for rimming the glass

Instructions:

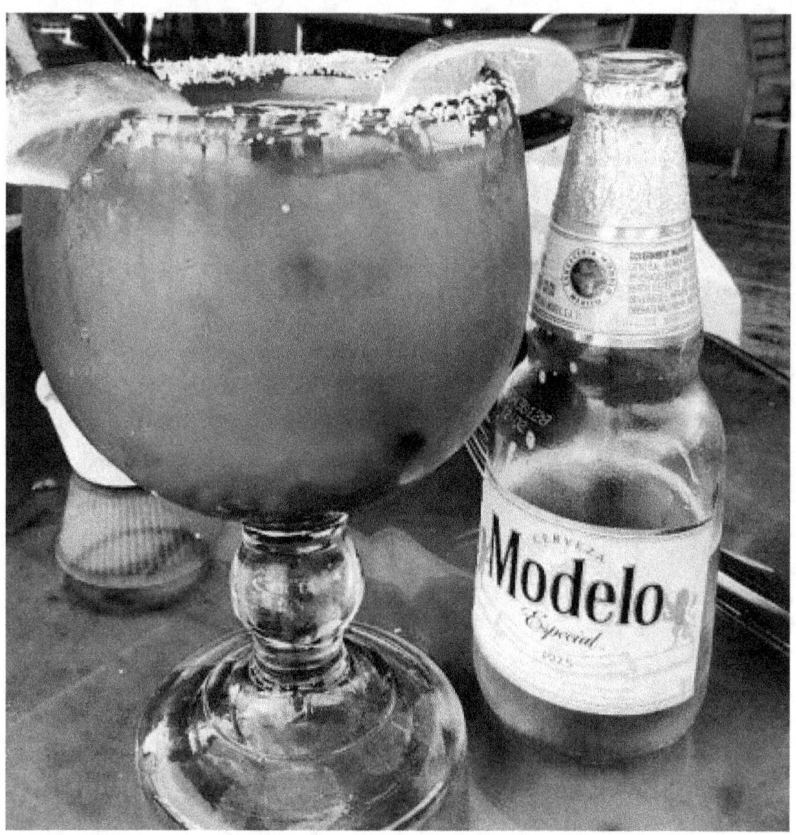

RIM A GLASS WITH SALT and chili powder.

Add lime juice, tomato juice, and sauces to the glass, then fill with ice.

Pour in the beer, stir gently, and enjoy!

Rompope

Rompope is a Mexican eggnog-like drink made with milk, sugar, egg yolks, and rum or brandy. This creamy, sweet drink is typically flavored with vanilla and cinnamon and is enjoyed around Christmas and other festive occasions.

How to Make Rompope
Ingredients:
4 cups of milk

1 cinnamon stick
1 cup sugar
6 egg yolks
1/2 cup of rum or brandy
1 tsp vanilla extract
Instructions:

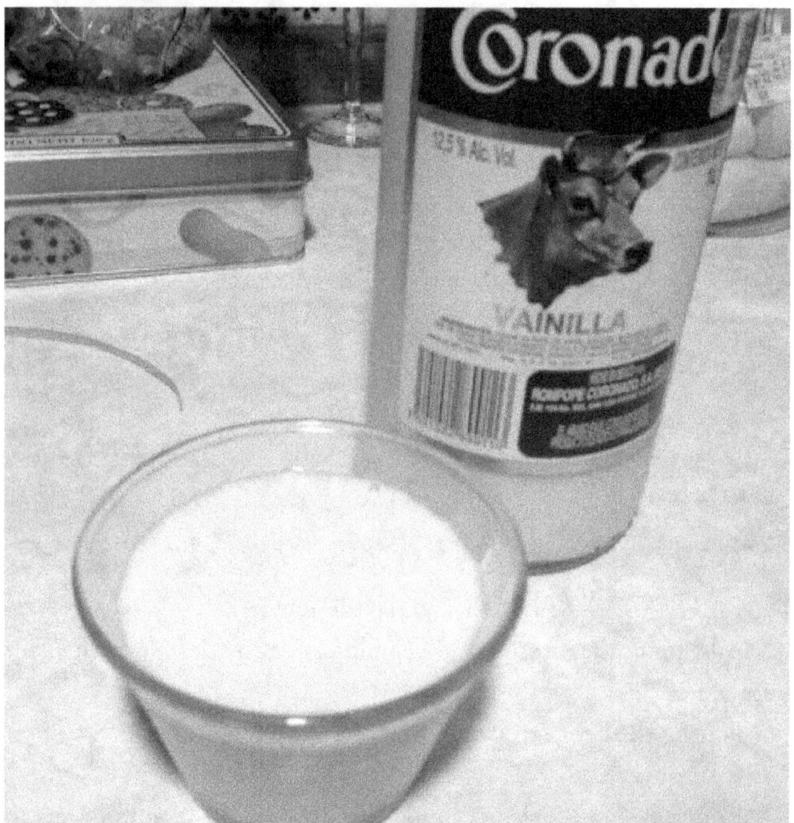

HEAT MILK, CINNAMON, and sugar in a saucepan. Simmer for 10 minutes.

In a separate bowl, whisk egg yolks. Slowly add the hot milk mixture to the eggs, stirring constantly.

Return the mixture to the pan and cook on low heat until thickened.

Remove from heat, add rum and vanilla, and chill before serving.

Champurrado

Champurrado is a chocolate-based version of atole, a thickened corn drink made with masa harina. It's a warm, comforting drink enjoyed during holidays and celebrations, often served with churros.

How to Make Champurrado

Ingredients:

4 cups of milk

1/4 cup masa harina

1-disc Mexican chocolate, chopped

1/4 cup piloncillo or brown sugar

1 cinnamon stick

Instructions:

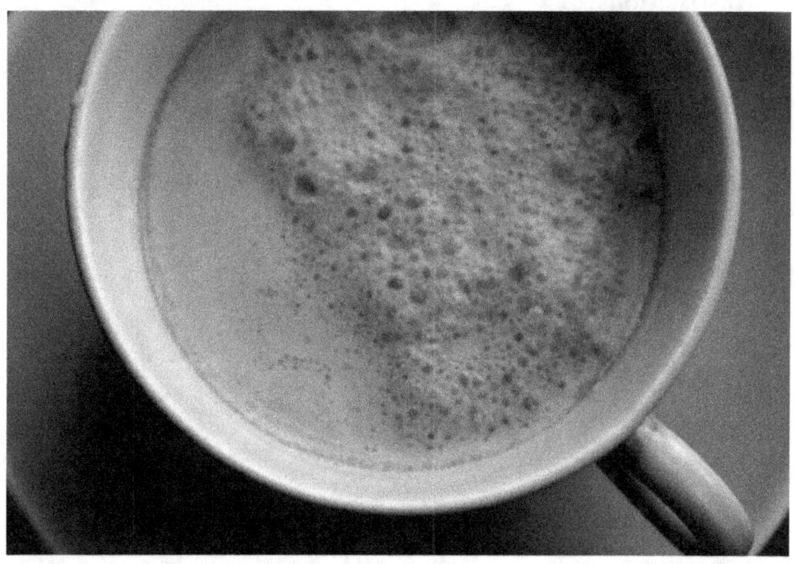

HEAT MILK IN A SAUCEPAN and add masa harina, stirring to dissolve.

Add the chocolate, piloncillo, and cinnamon stick, and cook over low heat until thickened.

Remove cinnamon stick and serve warm.

Café de Olla

Café de olla is a traditional Mexican coffee made with cinnamon and piloncillo, brewed in a clay pot (olla) that gives it a unique, earthy flavor. This sweet, spiced coffee is popular in rural areas and among coffee lovers looking for a unique twist on their morning brew.

How to Make Café de Olla

Ingredients:

4 cups of water

1 cinnamon stick

1/4 cup piloncillo or brown sugar

3 tbsp ground coffee

Instructions:

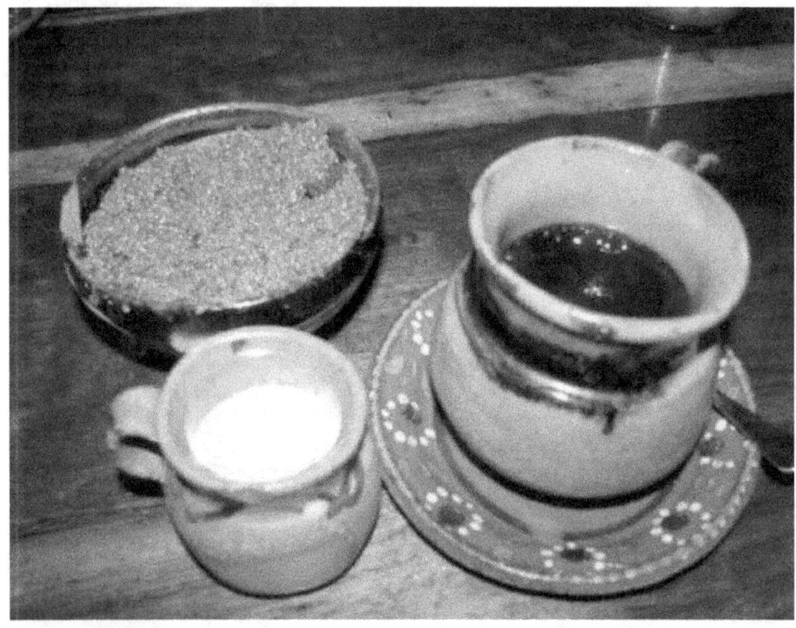

IN A POT, BOIL WATER with cinnamon and piloncillo until the sugar dissolves.

Add the coffee, simmer for a few minutes, then strain.

Serve hot for a deliciously spiced coffee experience.

Mexican drinks are as diverse and flavorful as the food, offering everything from refreshing aguas frescas and creamy horchata to bold mezcal and comforting champurrado. Each drink has its own story and regional variations, rooted in Mexico's rich cultural heritage. Whether you're sipping on a frothy mug of Mexican hot chocolate, cooling off with agua de tamarindo, or enjoying a shot of tequila, these beverages bring the spirit of Mexico to every glass. Try making these drinks at home for an authentic taste of Mexico's vibrant beverage culture.

1

Authentic Barbacoa Recipe

Barbacoa is a traditional Mexican dish that has been celebrated for centuries, known for its rich, savory flavor and melt-in-your-mouth tenderness. Traditionally made with lamb or beef, barbacoa is slowly cooked to perfection, absorbing the flavors of spices and herbs over hours. It's a favorite for gatherings and celebrations, often served with warm tortillas, fresh salsa, and chopped onions and cilantro. This authentic barbacoa recipe brings the taste of Mexico to your kitchen, preserving the essence of this beloved dish while making it accessible to cook at home.

Ingredients

4 lbs. beef cheeks or beef chuck roast (or lamb shoulder for a more traditional option)

4 garlic cloves, minced

1 large white onion, chopped

3-4 dried guajillo chiles

2 dried ancho chiles

1/4 cup of apple cider vinegar

1 tsp cumin

1/2 tsp ground cloves

1 tbsp dried oregano

2 bay leaves

Salt and pepper to taste

1 cup beef or chicken broth

2 tbsp vegetable oil (optional, for searing)

Fresh tortillas, chopped onions, cilantro, and lime for serving

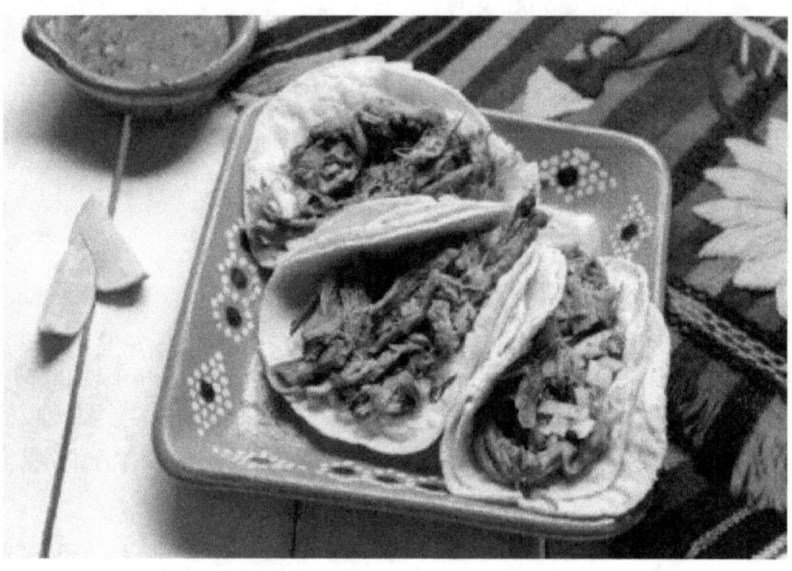

STEP-BY-STEP INSTRUCTIONS

1. Prepare the Chiles

Start by removing the stems and seeds from the dried guajillo and ancho chiles. In a small pot, bring water to a boil, then add the chiles and let them simmer for about 5 minutes or until they are softened. Drain the chiles and set them aside.

2. Make the Marinade

In a blender, combine the softened chiles, apple cider vinegar, minced garlic, cumin, ground cloves, oregano, and a pinch of salt and pepper. Add about half a cup of beef or chicken broth to help blend the ingredients into a smooth paste. This marinade is key to giving the barbacoa its authentic, deep flavor.

3. Marinate the Meat

Place the meat in a large bowl or a resealable plastic bag. Pour the marinade over the meat, ensuring it is fully coated. Let it marinate in the refrigerator for at least 4 hours, or preferably overnight, to allow the flavors to fully penetrate the meat.

4. Prepare for Cooking

Once the meat has marinated, preheat your oven to 275°F (135°C). If you prefer, you can sear the meat in a hot skillet with a bit of oil for a few minutes on each side to lock in the juices and add extra flavor.

5. Slow-Cook Meat

Transfer the marinated meat to a large, oven-safe pot with a lid (such as a Dutch oven). Add the chopped onion, bay leaves, and the remaining broth to the pot. Cover the pot with the lid and cook in the oven for 6-8 hours, or until the meat is tender and easily shreds with a fork.

Tip: If you don't have an oven-safe pot, you can use a slow cooker. Set it on low for 8-10 hours or high for 5-6 hours.

6. Shred the Meat

Once the meat is cooked, remove it from the pot and place it on a cutting board. Use two forks to shred the meat into bite-sized pieces. If there is excess liquid in the pot, you can add some back to the shredded meat to keep it moist and flavorful.

7. Serve and Enjoy

Your authentic barbacoa is ready to serve! Traditionally, it's enjoyed with warm corn tortillas, chopped onions, fresh cilantro, and a squeeze of lime. You can also add a splash of salsa or your favorite toppings.

Tips for Perfect Barbacoa

Use the Right Cut of Meat: For the best flavor and texture, opt for beef cheeks, beef chuck, or lamb shoulder. These cuts are well-marbled and break down beautifully during slow cooking.

Adjust the Spice: If you like more heat, you can add a few dried arbol chiles to the marinade or a pinch of crushed red pepper.

Resting Time: Letting the meat marinate overnight enhances its flavor, so don't skip this step if you have the time.

Serve Fresh: Barbacoa is best enjoyed right after it's cooked. However, leftovers can be stored in the refrigerator for up to 3 days or frozen for later use.

The History and Tradition of Barbacoa

Barbacoa dates to pre-Hispanic Mexico, where it was traditionally cooked in a pit covered with leaves, imparting a unique smoky flavor. This cooking method is still used in parts of Mexico today, especially for special occasions. Over time, barbacoa evolved to incorporate regional spices and methods, with each area adding its own twist.

The word "barbacoa" is the origin of "barbecue," though the methods and flavors differ greatly. What remains consistent is the emphasis on slow cooking and bold flavors that celebrate the rich culinary heritage of Mexico.

Why You'll Love This Recipe

Authentic barbacoa brings the taste of Mexico to your kitchen with every bite. It's a dish that's easy to prepare, yet its flavors are complex and rich, thanks to the slow-cooking process. Whether you're making it for a family gathering or a festive meal, barbacoa will impress everyone with its tender texture and depth of flavor.

Serve it in tacos, with rice and beans, or as the star of your favorite Mexican-inspired dishes. This barbacoa recipe will transport you to the heart of Mexico with every mouthful!

Creative Ways to Serve Barbacoa

One of the best things about barbacoa is its versatility! While traditionally served in tacos, barbacoa can be enjoyed in various ways. Here are a few ideas to get creative with your leftovers or add variety to your meal:

Barbacoa Tacos: Classic and delicious! Serve with warm corn tortillas, diced onions, cilantro, and a squeeze of lime for that authentic taco flavor.

Barbacoa Quesadillas: Place barbacoa and shredded cheese between two tortillas, then heat until golden and crispy. Serve with guacamole and salsa for a comforting snack.

Barbacoa Burrito Bowls: Skip the tortilla and pile barbacoa over a bed of rice with black beans, guacamole, pico de gallo, and shredded lettuce for a hearty bowl.

Barbacoa Tostadas: Spread refried beans over a crispy tostada shell, add a layer of barbacoa, and top with shredded lettuce, cheese, salsa, and a dollop of sour cream.

Barbacoa Enchiladas: Fill corn tortillas with barbacoa, roll them up, and place them in a baking dish. Cover with enchilada sauce, top with cheese, and bake until bubbly.

Barbacoa Soup: Use the leftover broth from cooking and add shredded barbacoa, some cooked potatoes, and vegetables like carrots and zucchini for a comforting soup.

Frequently Asked Questions about Barbacoa

Q: Can I make barbacoa in an Instant Pot?

Yes, if you're short on time, the Instant Pot is a great option for barbacoa. Sear the meat in the Instant Pot on the sauté setting, then add the marinade, spices, and broth. Cook on high pressure for 60-80 minutes (depending on the thickness of your meat) and allow for a natural pressure release. The result is a tender, flavorful barbacoa in a fraction of the time!

Q: What's the best way to store and reheat barbacoa?

Store any leftover barbacoa in an airtight container in the refrigerator for up to three days. For longer storage, freeze the meat in freezer-safe bags for up to three months. Reheat in a pot over low heat, adding a splash of water or broth to keep it moist.

Q: What side dishes pair well with barbacoa?

Barbacoa pairs well with classic Mexican sides like Mexican rice, refried beans, or charro beans. You can also serve it with roasted corn, grilled vegetables, or a fresh green salad. For a traditional feast, try it with homemade salsas, guacamole, and warm tortillas.

The Joy of Making Barbacoa at Home

Making barbacoa at home connects you to the rich traditions of Mexican cuisine. It's a dish that not only satisfies the taste buds but also celebrates the essence of slow-cooked, home-cooked meals. The process is one of patience and love, allowing the flavors to meld and develop into something truly special. Whether you're cooking for family or friends, barbacoa brings people together around the table, sharing the warmth and tradition of Mexican culture.

This authentic barbacoa recipe is perfect for those who enjoy exploring traditional dishes and savoring bold flavors. With a little preparation and time, you'll have a meal that's as rewarding to make as it is to enjoy. So, grab your ingredients, let the spices work their magic, and indulge in the rich, savory flavors of Mexican barbacoa—an unforgettable culinary experience!

2

Authentic Carne Asada Recipe

Carne Asada, or "grilled meat," is a staple in Mexican cuisine known for its smoky, charred flavors and succulent texture. Traditionally made with cuts like skirt or flank steak, carne asada is marinated in a blend of citrus, spices, and herbs, then grilled to perfection. It's a versatile dish that's enjoyed in tacos, burritos, or simply on its own with fresh salsas and tortillas. This recipe captures the authentic flavors of carne asada and brings the taste of Mexican street food right to your backyard grill!

Ingredients

2 lbs. skirt steak or flank steak

1/4 cup of orange juice

1/4 cup of lime juice (about 2-3 limes)

1/4 cup olive oil

3 cloves garlic, minced

1/4 cup fresh cilantro, chopped

1 tbsp soy sauce

1 tbsp Worcestershire sauce

1 tsp ground cumin

1 tsp chili powder

Salt and pepper, to taste

Fresh tortillas, chopped onions, cilantro, and lime wedges for serving

Step-by-Step Instructions

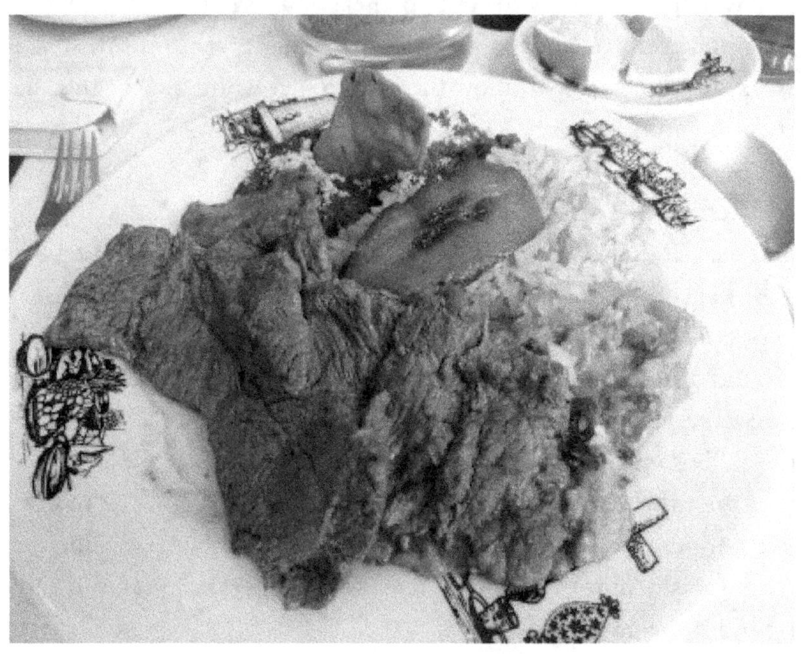

1. PREPARE THE MARINADE

In a mixing bowl, combine orange juice, lime juice, olive oil, minced garlic, chopped cilantro, soy sauce, Worcestershire sauce, cumin, and chili powder. Whisk everything together until it is well combined. This marinade is what gives carne asada its signature flavor with a balance of acidity, spice, and herbal notes.

2. Marinate the Steak

Place the skirt or flank steak in a large resealable plastic bag or shallow dish. Pour the marinade over the steak, ensuring it's fully coated. Seal the bag or cover the dish, then let the steak marinate in the refrigerator for at least 2 hours, or up to 8 hours for the best flavor. The citrus juices tenderize the meat, making it juicy and flavorful after grilling.

3. Prepare the Grill

When you're ready to cook, preheat your grill to high heat. You want the grill to be hot to achieve a nice char on the outside of the steak. If using charcoal, allow the coals to get white-hot for that authentic smoky flavor.

4. Grill the Steak

Remove the steak from the marinade, letting any excess drip off, and place it directly on the hot grill. Cook for about 3-5 minutes per side, depending on the thickness of the steak and your desired level of doneness. For medium-rare, aim for an internal temperature of around 130-135°F. Skirt and flank steak are best cooked medium-rare to keep them tender and juicy.

5. Rest and Slice

Once the steak is done, remove it from the grill and let it rest for 5-10 minutes. Resting allows the juices to redistribute, keeping the steak moist. After resting, slice the steak against the grain into thin strips for the most tender texture.

6. Serve and Enjoy

Serve the carne asada with warm tortillas, a sprinkle of chopped onions and cilantro, and a squeeze of fresh lime juice. Add some salsa or guacamole for an extra burst of flavor. Carne asada can be served in tacos, burritos, or even in a bowl with rice and beans for a complete meal.

Tips for Perfect Carne Asada

Choosing the Right Cut: Skirt steak and flank steak are traditional choices for carne asada due to their rich flavor and relatively quick cooking time. These cuts absorb marinades well and develop a great char when grilled.

Marinate for Maximum Flavor: Letting the meat marinate for at least 2 hours allows the citrus and spices to penetrate the steak, resulting in a more flavorful dish.

Grill Temperature: Use high heat to get a nice char on the steak. This sears the outside, locking in the juices and enhancing the smoky flavor.

Slice Against the Grain: Cutting the steak against the grain shortens the muscle fibers, making the meat more tender and easier to chew.

Serving Suggestions and Side Dishes

Carne asada is incredibly versatile, and there are countless ways to enjoy it. Here are a few serving ideas and sides to completing your meal:

Carne Asada Tacos: Serve the carne asada in warm corn tortillas with chopped onions, cilantro, and your favorite salsa.

Carne Asada Burritos: Wrap the sliced carne asada in a flour tortilla with rice, beans, cheese, and guacamole.

Carne Asada Nachos: Top tortilla chips with sliced carne asada, melted cheese, pico de gallo, guacamole, and jalapeños for a hearty snack or meal.

Carne Asada Fries: Layer French fries with carne asada, cheese, and your favorite toppings for an indulgent treat.

Classic Sides: Pair your carne asada with Mexican rice, refried beans, grilled corn, or a fresh salad for a complete meal.

The Cultural Roots of Carne Asada

Carne asada is more than just a dish—it's a celebration of Mexican grilling culture. In Mexico, carne asada is often the centerpiece of family gatherings and outdoor parties, called "asados" or "parrilladas." Friends and family come together to share good food, conversation, and time-honored recipes. The smoky, charred flavors of carne asada capture the essence of communal cooking, where the grill is a place to connect with others over delicious food.

While every region and family may have its own twist on the marinade or preparation, the core of carne asada remains the same:

simple, fresh ingredients, carefully marinated meat, and the unmistakable flavor of a hot grill.

Frequently Asked Questions

Q: Can I cook carne asada on a stovetop if I don't have a grill?

Yes! If you don't have a grill, you can cook carne asada on a cast-iron skillet or grill pan. Heat the pan over high heat until it's very hot, then cook the steak as you would on a grill. You won't get the same smoky flavor, but you'll still achieve a great char and delicious taste.

Q: How long should I marinate the carne asada?

While 2 hours is the minimum recommended time, marinating for 4-8 hours will give you the best flavor. However, avoid marinating for more than 12 hours, as the citrus can break down the meat too much and affect the texture.

Q: What if my steak is tough?

If you find that your steak is tough, ensure you're slicing against the grain. This is crucial for skirt and flank steak as it shortens the muscle fibers, making the meat more tender. Also, avoid overcooking, as these cuts can become chewy when cooked past medium.

Why You'll Love Authentic Carne Asada

Authentic carne asada offers bold, zesty flavors with minimal ingredients. The beauty of this dish lies in its simplicity and versatility. From its tender, juicy slices to its smoky charred exterior, carne asada brings the taste of Mexico's street food right to your table. It's perfect for casual dinners, taco nights, or summer cookouts, offering a vibrant experience with every bite. Whether you're preparing it for a small family dinner or a large gathering, carne asada is a surefire crowd-pleaser. With its rich marinade, high-heat grilling, and simple yet flavorful presentation, this recipe will make you feel like a true grill master, capturing the spirit of Mexican cooking in your own home.

3

Authentic Chalupa Recipe

Chalupas are a delicious Mexican street food originating from Puebla, known for their crispy texture and rich toppings. Made from small, thick corn tortillas fried until crispy, chalupas are typically topped with ingredients like shredded meat, salsa, cheese, and lettuce, creating a flavorful and satisfying bite-sized dish. This recipe captures the authenticity of Mexican chalupas, offering a delightful combination of textures and flavors.

Ingredients

For the Chalupa Base:

1 1/2 cups masa harina (corn flour)

1 cup warm water (adjust as needed)

A pinch of salt

Vegetable oil for frying

For the Toppings:

1/2 lb. cooked shredded beef, pork, or chicken

1 cup salsa verde or salsa roja (green or red salsa)

1/2 cup crumbled queso fresco or grated cotija cheese

1/2 cup of shredded lettuce

1/4 cup chopped onions (optional)

Fresh cilantro for garnish

Lime wedges for serving

Step-by-Step Instructions

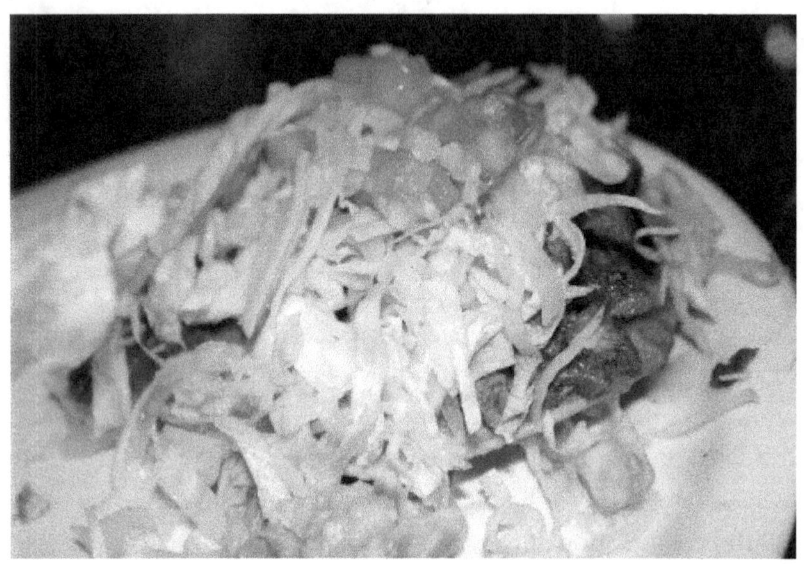

1. MAKE THE MASA DOUGH

In a mixing bowl, combine the masa harina and salt. Gradually add warm water, mixing with your hands until the dough comes together. It should be smooth and pliable, like playdough in texture. If it feels too dry, add a bit more water; if it's too sticky, sprinkle in a bit more masa harina.

2. Shape the Chalupas

Divide the dough into small balls, about the size of a golf ball. Flatten each ball between your hands or with a tortilla press until they form thick, small discs around 3-4 inches in diameter. These discs will be the base of your chalupas and should be slightly thicker than a regular tortilla to hold the toppings well.

3. Fry the Chalupas

In a skillet, heat about 1/4 inch of vegetable oil over medium heat. Once the oil is hot (you can test by dropping a small piece of dough if it sizzles, it's ready), carefully place a few of the masa discs into the oil. Fry for 2-3 minutes on each side or until golden and crispy. Transfer them to a paper towel-lined plate to drain excess oil. Repeat until all the chalupa bases are fried.

4. Add the Toppings

Once the chalupa bases are fried, it's time to add your toppings. Spread a spoonful of salsa over each chalupa, covering the surface. Top with shredded meat (beef, pork, or chicken works well), a sprinkle of crumbled queso fresco or cotija cheese, and some shredded lettuce. You can also add chopped onions and fresh cilantro if you like.

5. Serve and Enjoy

Arrange the chalupas on a platter, garnish with fresh cilantro, and serve with lime wedges on the side. Chalupas are best enjoyed fresh and warm, with a squeeze of lime juice for added brightness.

Tips for Perfect Chalupas

Use Fresh Masa: For the best flavor, use masa harina specifically made for tortillas. Fresh masa harina gives chalupas an authentic taste and texture.

Adjust the Thickness: Chalupa bases should be thicker than a typical tortilla but not too thick. This thickness helps them stay crispy while holding the toppings without getting soggy.

Keep the Oil Hot: To get that perfect crispy texture, make sure your oil is consistently hot. Lower temperatures can cause the chalupas to absorb more oil, making them greasy.

Customize Your Toppings: While traditional chalupas often use shredded meat and salsa, you can get creative. Try adding guacamole, refried beans, or even a drizzle of sour cream for a unique twist.

Traditional Versus Restaurant-Style Chalupas

In Mexico, chalupas are typically smaller and made with simple toppings, focusing on high-quality ingredients like fresh salsa and cheese. They differ from the larger, more elaborate versions often found in restaurants or fast-food chains. The authentic chalupas are all about balance, allowing the crispy base, fresh salsa, and toppings to shine without overwhelming flavors.

Serving Suggestions and Pairings

Chalupas are perfect for gatherings and can be served as appetizers, snacks, or even a main dish if you offer a few per person. To round out the meal, you can pair chalupas with classic Mexican sides like:

Refried Beans: Creamy and flavorful, refried beans make a perfect side dish.

Mexican Rice: Lightly seasoned rice is a great accompaniment for chalupas, balancing their flavors.

Fresh Salsa and Guacamole: Serve with extra salsa and guacamole for dipping.

Mexican Elote (Street Corn): Grilled corn topped with mayonnaise, cheese, and spices adds a fun and delicious option to your chalupa spread.

The Cultural Roots of Chalupas

Chalupas hold a special place in Mexican street food culture, especially in the central and southern regions like Puebla. They're a common sight at street stalls and markets, with each vendor adding their own twist, from the type of salsa to the toppings used. Chalupas showcase Mexico's vibrant culinary heritage, offering a delicious snapshot of its diverse flavors and cooking techniques.

Frequently Asked Questions

Q: Can I bake the chalupas instead of frying them?

Yes, you can bake them if you prefer a lighter version. Brush each chalupa base with a bit of oil, place them on a baking sheet, and bake at 400°F (200°C) for about 10-12 minutes or until golden and crispy.

Q: What's the difference between chalupas and tostadas?

While similar, chalupas and tostadas have a few differences. Chalupas are typically thicker, and their dough may be slightly thicker to support the toppings. Tostadas are usually made with a thinner, flat tortilla that's fried until crisp. Both are delicious but offer different textures and topping options.

Q: Can I make chalupa bases in advance?

Yes, you can prepare the chalupa bases a day in advance. Store them in an airtight container at room temperature. To reheat, place them in a hot oven or lightly pan-fry for a few minutes to restore their crispiness.

Why You'll Love This Authentic Chalupa Recipe

Authentic chalupas are simple, delicious, and packed with traditional Mexican flavors. They're perfect for gatherings or family meals, offering a fun, interactive way to enjoy classic ingredients in a new form. The combination of the crispy chalupa base with fresh salsa, tender meat, and vibrant toppings creates a satisfying dish that's hard to resist. With their rich history and crowd-pleasing flavors, chalupas are a wonderful way to bring Mexican street food into your kitchen. So, gather your ingredients, heat up your skillet, and enjoy a taste of Mexico with these authentic, delicious chalupas!

4

Authentic Chicken Enchilada Recipe

Chicken enchiladas are a classic Mexican dish that brings together tender, shredded chicken, rich red enchilada sauce, and soft corn tortillas, all baked to perfection with melted cheese on top. Enchiladas are hearty, comforting, and burst with flavor, making them a popular meal for family gatherings and celebrations. This authentic recipe keeps it simple, focusing on traditional ingredients that capture the essence of Mexican home cooking.

Ingredients

For the Chicken Filling:

2 lbs. chicken breast or thighs, cooked and shredded

1 small onion, finely chopped

2 garlic cloves, minced

1 tbsp vegetable oil

Salt and pepper to taste

For the Red Enchilada Sauce:

4-5 dried guajillo chiles

1-2 dried ancho chiles

2 cups of chicken broth

1 tbsp tomato paste

2 garlic cloves

1/2 tsp ground cumin

1/2 tsp dried oregano

Salt to taste

For Assembly:

12-15 corn tortillas

1 cup shredded queso fresco or Monterrey Jack cheese (or a mix)
Fresh cilantro, chopped, for garnish
Sliced green onions and sour cream for topping (optional)
Step-by-Step Instructions

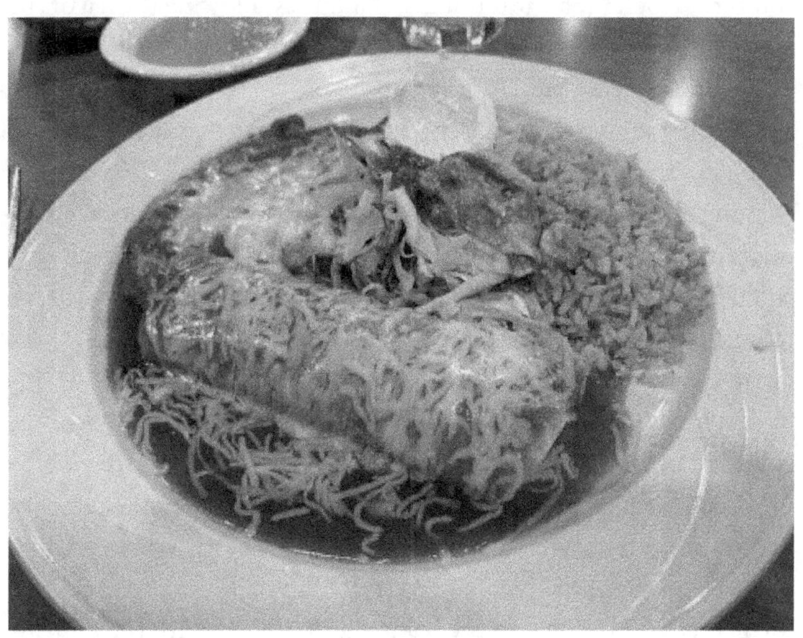

1. PREPARE THE ENCHILADA Sauce

Remove the stems and seeds from the guajillo and ancho chiles. In a small pot, bring water to a boil, then add the chiles and simmer for about 5 minutes, or until they're softened. Drain the chiles and place them in a blender with chicken broth, tomato paste, garlic, cumin, oregano, and a pinch of salt. Blend until smooth.

Pour the sauce into a skillet and bring it to a simmer over medium heat. Let it cook for 5-10 minutes until it thickens slightly, then adjust the salt to taste. The sauce should be vibrant and flavorful, with a rich, deep red color. Set aside.

2. Cook the Chicken Filling

In a skillet, heat the vegetable oil over medium heat. Add the chopped onion and cook until translucent, for about 5 minutes. Add the minced garlic and cook for another minute, until fragrant. Add the shredded chicken, season with salt and pepper, and stir well to combine. Cook for an additional 2-3 minutes, allowing the flavors to meld. Set the chicken filling aside.

3. Prepare the Corn Tortillas

Authentic enchiladas use corn tortillas, which need a little preparation to prevent them from breaking when rolled. Heat a small amount of oil in a skillet over medium heat. Quickly pass each tortilla through the oil for a few seconds on each side, just until softened. This step also adds flavor and helps the tortillas absorb the sauce. Place the tortillas on paper towels to absorb excess oil.

4. Assemble the Enchiladas

Preheat your oven to 375°F (190°C). Pour a small amount of enchilada sauce into the bottom of a baking dish to prevent sticking.

Take one softened tortilla, dip it lightly in the enchilada sauce, and place it on a plate. Spoon a small amount of the chicken filling onto the center of the tortilla, then roll it up tightly. Place the rolled tortilla seam-side down in the baking dish. Repeat with the remaining tortillas and chicken filling, arranging them snugly in the dish.

5. Add Sauce and Cheese

Pour the remaining enchilada sauce over the rolled enchiladas, ensuring they are well-coated. Sprinkle the shredded cheese evenly over the top.

6. Bake the Enchiladas

Cover the baking dish with aluminum foil and bake it in the preheated oven for about 20 minutes. Remove the foil and bake for an additional 5-10 minutes, or until the cheese is melted, bubbly, and slightly golden.

7. Garnish and Serve

Once the enchiladas are done, remove them from the oven and let them cool slightly. Garnish with fresh cilantro, green onions, and a dollop of sour cream if desired. Serve hot with a side of Mexican rice, refried beans, or a simple green salad.

Tips for Perfect Chicken Enchiladas

Use Good Quality Chiles: Dried guajillo and ancho chiles add authentic flavor and color to the sauce. Look for soft, pliable chiles for the best results.

Choose the Right Tortillas: Corn tortillas are traditional for enchiladas. If possible, use fresh, high-quality tortillas that won't tear when rolled.

Control the Sauce Consistency: Your sauce should be thick enough to cling to the enchiladas but not too thick. Add a bit more broth if needed to reach the right consistency. Layer for Flavor: Dipping each tortilla in sauce before rolling helps infuse the enchiladas with flavor from the inside out.

Variations and Serving Suggestions

Chicken enchiladas are delicious on their own, but you can also try variations to suit your taste:

Add Beans: Mix a bit of refried or black beans into the chicken filling for extra heartiness.

Top with Fresh Ingredients: Garnish with avocado slices, jalapeños, or a sprinkle of cotija cheese for extra flavor.

Serve with Traditional Sides: Enchiladas pair beautifully with sides like Mexican rice, refried beans, or grilled corn on the cob.

The History and Tradition of Enchiladas

Enchiladas date back to the Aztecs, who wrap small fish in tortillas and enjoy them with a variety of sauces. Over time, enchiladas evolved to include different fillings and sauces, making them a versatile dish enjoyed in various forms across Mexico. Authentic enchiladas are simple yet deeply flavorful, celebrating the beauty of corn tortillas, chiles, and fresh ingredients.

Frequently Asked Questions

Q: Can I make the enchilada sauce in advance?

Yes, the sauce can be made ahead and stored in the refrigerator for up to 3 days. Simply reheat it on the stove before using it.

Q: What's the difference between enchiladas and burritos?

Enchiladas are made with corn tortillas, filled with ingredients, and covered in sauce, then baked. Burritos are typically made with large flour tortillas, filled, and often served without sauce.

Q: Can I use store-bought enchilada sauce?

While homemade sauce offers the best flavor, you can use a high-quality store-bought enchilada sauce if you're short on time.

Why You'll Love This Authentic Chicken Enchilada Recipe

Authentic chicken enchiladas are a celebration of flavor, texture, and tradition. The combination of tender chicken, smoky red sauce, and melted cheese wrapped in soft corn tortillas makes for a dish that's both comforting and satisfying. Whether you're making them for a family dinner or a festive gathering, chicken enchiladas bring warmth and a taste of Mexican culture to your table. With just a few key ingredients and simple steps, you'll be able to recreate these delicious enchiladas in your own kitchen. Serve them with classic Mexican sides and let the flavors transport you straight to the heart of Mexico!

5

Authentic Chicken Fajitas Recipe

Chicken fajitas are a beloved Mexican dish known for their sizzling presentation and vibrant flavors. Made with marinated chicken, colorful bell peppers, onions, and a mix of spices, fajitas are served hot off the grill or skillet, ready to be wrapped in warm tortillas with your favorite toppings. This recipe captures the authentic essence of chicken fajitas, combining traditional ingredients with simple techniques for a dish that's perfect for weeknight dinners or gatherings.

Ingredients

For the Marinade:

2 lbs. boneless, skinless chicken breasts or thighs, sliced into strips

1/4 cup olive oil

1/4 cup of lime juice (about 2-3 limes)

3 garlic cloves, minced

1 tsp ground cumin

1 tsp chili powder

1 tsp smoked paprika

1/2 tsp oregano

1/2 tsp salt

1/4 tsp black pepper

For the Fajitas:

1 red bell pepper, sliced

1 green bell pepper, sliced

1 yellow bell pepper, sliced

1 large onion, sliced

2 tbsp vegetable oil for cooking

Warm flour or corn tortillas for serving

Optional Toppings:

Guacamole

Salsa

Sour cream

Shredded cheese

Fresh cilantro

Lime wedges

Step-by-Step Instructions

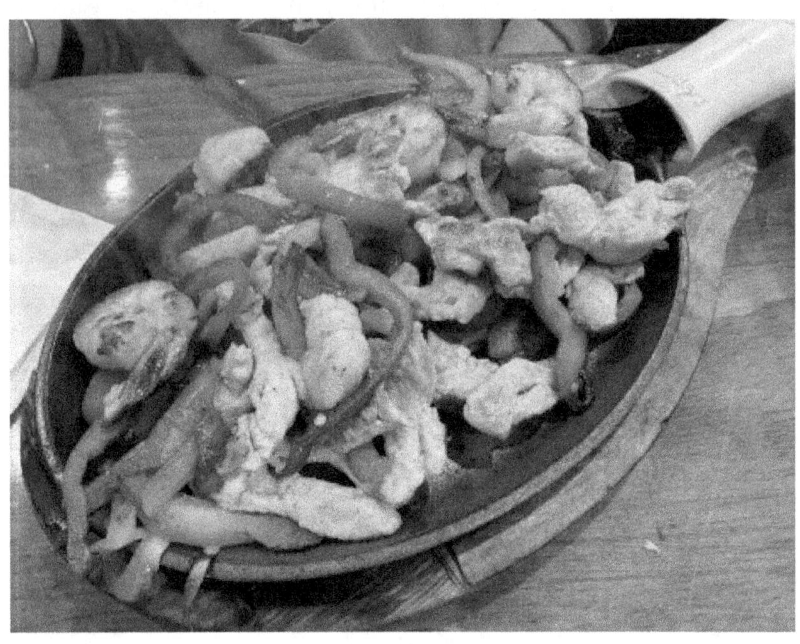

1. MARINATE THE CHICKEN

In a large bowl, whisk together olive oil, lime juice, minced garlic, cumin, chili powder, smoked paprika, oregano, salt, and pepper
to create the marinade. Add the sliced chicken to the bowl and toss

to coat evenly. Cover and refrigerate for at least 30 minutes, but preferably for 1-2 hours to allow the flavors to fully develop.

Tip: Marinating the chicken in lime juice adds brightness and tenderizes the meat, resulting in juicy and flavorful fajitas.

2. Cook the Vegetables

Heat 1 tablespoon of vegetable oil in a large skillet or cast-iron pan over medium-high heat. Add the sliced bell peppers and onions, and cook for 5-7 minutes, stirring occasionally, until they become tender and slightly charred around the edges. Once cooked, transfer the vegetables to a plate and set aside.

3. Cook the Chicken

In the same skillet, heat the remaining tablespoon of vegetable oil over medium-high heat. Add the marinated chicken strips to the pan in a single layer. Cook the chicken for 5-6 minutes per side, or until it's fully cooked and lightly browned. The chicken should reach an internal temperature of 165°F (75°C).

4. Combine and Serve

Once the chicken is cooked through, return the sautéed peppers and onions to the skillet. Stir everything together to combine and heat for another 2-3 minutes. Remove the skillet from the heat.

Serve the chicken fajitas sizzling hot with warm tortillas on the side. Let everyone assemble their fajitas with their preferred toppings like guacamole, salsa, sour cream, shredded cheese, and fresh cilantro.

Tips for Perfect Chicken Fajitas

Use the Right Pan: A cast-iron skillet or grill pan works best for fajitas because it retains heat well and helps create a nice sear on the chicken and vegetables.

Don't Overcrowd the Pan: When cooking the chicken and vegetables, avoid overcrowding the pan to ensure even cooking and proper browning.

Marinate for Maximum Flavor: The marinade is key to flavorful fajitas. If you have the time, marinate the chicken for 2 hours or even overnight to enhance the flavors.

Keep It Sizzling: Serve fajitas straight from the skillet for that classic sizzling presentation. You can place the skillet on a heat-safe trivet in the center of the table for a fun, interactive dining experience.

Variations of Chicken Fajitas

While traditional chicken fajitas are made with a combination of bell peppers, onions, and seasoned chicken, there are many ways to customize this dish to your taste:

Add Extra Veggies: Try adding sliced zucchini, mushrooms, or tomatoes for more variety.

Use Different Proteins: Fajitas can also be made with beef, shrimp, or a combination of proteins for a mixed fajita platter.

Spice It Up: For those who like heat, add a few slices of jalapeños or a sprinkle of cayenne pepper to the marinade.

Traditional Fajitas vs. Restaurant-Style Fajitas

Authentic fajitas, originating from Northern Mexico and Texas (Tex-Mex cuisine), were traditionally made with skirt steak, marinated, and grilled, then served with vegetables. Over time, chicken fajitas became just as popular, and the dish has evolved into the sizzling version often seen at Mexican restaurants today.

In its most traditional form, fajitas are all about simplicity—grilled meat, vegetables, and tortillas. However, restaurant-style fajitas often include more elaborate toppings like cheese, sour cream, and guacamole. Both versions are delicious, but authentic fajitas focus on the flavors of the marinade and the freshness of the ingredients.

Serving Suggestions

Chicken fajitas are versatile and can be served in many ways. Here are a few ideas to complete your fajita meal:

Side of Rice and Beans: Serve with Mexican rice and refried beans or black beans for a classic pairing.

Fresh Salad: A simple side salad with lettuce, tomatoes, and avocado complements the fajitas and adds freshness to the meal.

Tortilla Chips and Salsa: Start with a bowl of tortilla chips, salsa, and guacamole as an appetizer to set the stage for the main event.

The History of Fajitas

Fajitas have their roots in Northern Mexico and the Southwestern United States, specifically in the ranching culture along the Texas-Mexico border. Originally, fajitas (derived from the Spanish word "faja," meaning "belt" or "strip") were made with skirt steak, a tough cut of meat that was marinated and grilled to make it tender and flavorful. The dish gained popularity in the 1930s and 1940s, when it was served by Mexican ranch workers. Over time, it evolved into the sizzling, restaurant-style fajitas we know today, with chicken, shrimp, and even vegetarian versions becoming popular options.

Frequently Asked Questions

Q: Can I cook chicken fajitas on the grill

Yes! Grilling adds a smoky flavor that enhances the fajitas. Marinate the chicken as instructed, then grill the chicken and vegetables over medium-high heat until they're charred and cooked through. Slice the grilled chicken and serve with the vegetables.

Q: What's the difference between fajitas and tacos?

Fajitas are typically served with grilled meats and vegetables that are assembled in tortillas, while tacos can be filled with a variety of ingredients and are often served with a wider range of toppings. Fajitas are usually served in a skillet, allowing diners to create their own wraps.

Q: Can I make fajitas ahead of time?

You can prepare the chicken and vegetable mixture ahead of time, store it in the refrigerator, and reheat it just before serving.

However, fajitas are best served fresh for that signature sizzling effect.

Why You'll Love This Authentic Chicken Fajitas Recipe

Chicken fajitas are quick, easy, and packed with bold, fresh flavors. The zesty marinade infuses the chicken with tangy lime and spices, while the sautéed bell peppers and onions add sweetness and crunch. Served with warm tortillas and your favorite toppings, chicken fajitas make for a fun, interactive meal that everyone can customize to their liking. Whether you're preparing a weeknight dinner or hosting a casual gathering, this authentic chicken fajita recipe is sure to impress. The combination of juicy chicken, colorful veggies, and a sizzling presentation makes it a flavorful and satisfying dish that's loved by all ages. Enjoy the taste of Mexico right in your own kitchen!

6

Authentic Chimichanga Recipe

Chimichangas are a beloved Tex-Mex dish known for their golden, crispy exterior and flavorful, savory fillings. Essentially a deep-fried burrito, chimichangas are packed with seasoned meat, rice, beans, and cheese, creating a delicious hearty meal that's both satisfying and fun. While they may not be traditional Mexican fare, chimichangas are a popular choice across the Southwest and beyond. This recipe will show you how to make restaurant-quality chimichangas right in your own kitchen.

Ingredients

For the Filling:

1 lb. shredded cooked chicken, beef, or pork

1/2 cup of cooked rice (optional)

1/2 cup of refried beans (optional)

1/2 cup shredded cheese (Monterey Jack or cheddar work well)

1 small onion, finely chopped

1 bell pepper, chopped

2 garlic cloves, minced

1 tbsp vegetable oil

1 tsp ground cumin

1 tsp chili powder

Salt and pepper to taste

For the Chimichangas:

6 large flour tortillas

Oil for frying (vegetable or canola oil)

Toothpicks (to secure the chimichangas)

For Serving:
Shredded lettuce
Pico de gallo
Sour cream
Guacamole
Salsa
Fresh cilantro for garnish
Step-by-Step Instructions

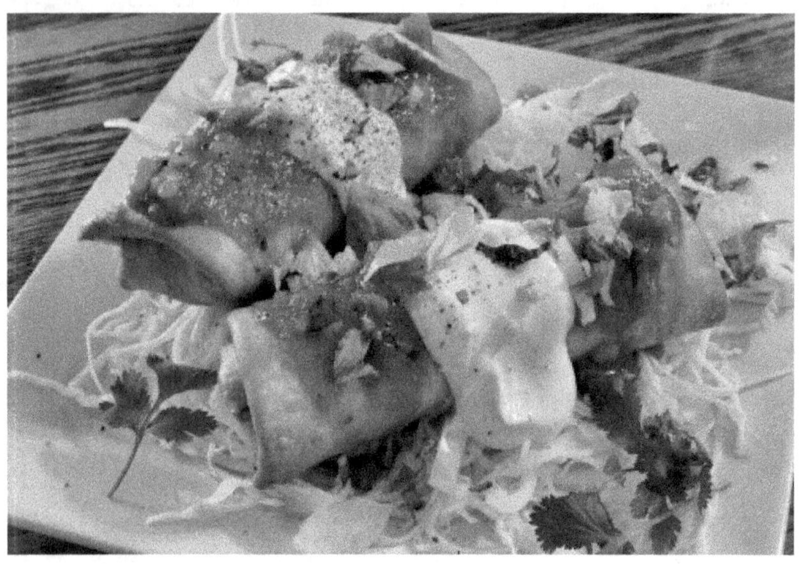

1. PREPARE THE FILLING

In a large skillet, heat the vegetable oil over medium heat. Add the chopped onion and bell pepper, and cook for about 5 minutes, or until the onion is translucent and the peppers are tender. Add the minced garlic and cook for another minute until fragrant.

Add the shredded meat (chicken, beef, or pork) to the skillet, along with cumin, chili powder, salt, and pepper. Stir well to combine and heat the mixture for another 5-7 minutes, allowing the flavors to meld together. Once the meat is warmed through, remove the skillet from the heat and set it aside.

If desired, mix in the cooked rice, refried beans, and shredded cheese to create a hearty, creamy filling for your chimichangas.

2. Assemble the Chimichangas

Lay a flour tortilla flat on a clean surface. Spoon about 1/3 cup of the filling mixture into the center of the tortilla. Fold the sides of the tortilla in toward the center, then fold up the bottom and roll tightly, securing the chimichanga with a toothpick if needed. Repeat with the remaining tortillas and filling.

Tip: Be careful not to overfill the tortillas, as they can burst while frying. Keep the filling amount moderate to ensure a secure roll.

3. Fry the Chimichangas

In a deep skillet or large pot, heat about 1 inch of vegetable oil over medium-high heat. To check if the oil is ready, place a small piece of tortilla in the oil; if it sizzles and bubbles, the oil is ready for frying.

Carefully place the assembled chimichangas in the hot oil, seam-side down, and fry for about 2-3 minutes per side, or until golden brown and crispy. Use tongs to turn the chimichangas, ensuring even frying on all sides. Once done, transfer the chimichangas to a paper towel-lined plate to drain excess oil.

Alternative Option: If you prefer a lighter version, brush the assembled chimichangas with oil and bake them in a preheated oven at 400°F (200°C) for 20-25 minutes, flipping halfway through until crispy and golden.

4. Serve and Garnish

Place the fried chimichangas on a serving plate. Top with shredded lettuce, a dollop of sour cream, a spoonful of pico de gallo, and guacamole. You can also drizzle salsa or melted cheese on top for an extra burst of flavor. Garnish with fresh cilantro and enjoy!

Tips for Perfect Chimichangas

Secure the Tortilla: Make sure the tortilla is tightly wrapped around the filling and use toothpicks to keep it in place if needed. This will help prevent it from opening during frying.

Avoid Overcrowding: Fry the chimichangas in batches if necessary to prevent them from sticking together and to maintain an even temperature in the oil.

Try Different Fillings: Chimichangas are versatile and can be customized with different fillings, such as ground beef, shrimp, or vegetables for a vegetarian option.

Chimichangas vs. Burritos

While chimichangas and burritos share similar ingredients, the key difference is that chimichangas are deep-fried, giving them a crispy, golden exterior. Burritos are typically served soft and not fried. Chimichangas also tend to include toppings like lettuce, sour cream, and salsa on top, while burritos are often served with toppings inside the tortilla.

Serving Suggestions and Sides

Chimichangas are a filling dish on their own, but you can serve them with sides to create a complete Tex-Mex-inspired meal:

Mexican Rice: Lightly seasoned rice adds a nice balance to the rich chimichangas.

Refried Beans: Creamy and flavorful, refried beans are a classic accompaniment.

Elote (Mexican Street Corn): Grilled corn topped with cheese, mayo, and chili powder is a great side.

Fresh Salsa and Guacamole: Serve with extra salsa and guacamole on the side for dipping.

The History of Chimichangas

Chimichangas originated in the Southwestern United States, particularly in Arizona and Texas, where they have become a beloved Tex-Mex specialty. Legend has it that the chimichanga was accidentally invented when a burrito was dropped into a flyer, and the result was so delicious it became a staple on menus throughout the region. Though the story of its origin varies, the chimichanga's crispy texture and savory filling have made it a favorite across borders.

Frequently Asked Questions

Q: Can I make chimichangas with a different type of meat?

Absolutely! Beef, pork, shrimp, or even vegetarian fillings like beans and grilled vegetables all work well in chimichangas. The key is to use a filling that's not too moist, as this helps keep the tortilla crispy.

Q: Are chimichangas always fried?

Traditionally, yes, but you can also bake them for a lighter option. Simply brush the assembled chimichangas with oil and bake at 400°F (200°C) for 20-25 minutes, turning halfway for even crisping.

Q: What's the best way to reheat chimichangas?

To keep chimichangas crispy, reheat them in an oven at 350°F (175°C) for about 10 minutes. Avoid microwaving, as it can make the tortilla soggy.

Why You'll Love This Authentic Chimichanga Recipe

Chimichangas are the perfect combination of crispy, cheesy, and savory. With a golden, crunchy tortilla shell and a flavorful, tender filling, they're the ultimate comfort food that's as fun to make as it is to eat. Whether you're looking for a new Tex-Mex recipe to try or want to recreate a favorite restaurant at home, this authentic chimichanga recipe delivers all the satisfying flavors you crave. Served with fresh toppings and your favorite Tex-Mex sides, chimichangas make a fantastic meal that's ideal for family dinners, parties, or simply treating yourself to something deliciously indulgent. Enjoy the crispy goodness of homemade chimichangas and savor every bite of this Tex-Mex classic!

7

Authentic Frijoles Refritos Recipe

Traditional Mexican Refried Beans

Frijoles Refritos, or refried beans, are a classic Mexican dish that adds creamy texture, rich flavor, and versatility to any meal. Despite the name, "refritos" doesn't mean "refried"; it translates to "well-fried" in Spanish. Authentic frijoles refritos are cooked and mashed pinto beans, often cooked in lard or oil and seasoned to perfection. This recipe will guide you through making authentic Mexican refried beans that are creamy, flavorful, and easy to make at home.

Ingredients

1 lb. dried pinto beans

6 cups of water (for cooking the beans)

1/4 cup of lard or vegetable oil (for a vegetarian option)

1 small white onion, finely chopped

2 garlic cloves, minced

Salt to taste

Optional toppings: crumbled queso fresco, chopped fresh cilantro

Step-by-Step Instructions

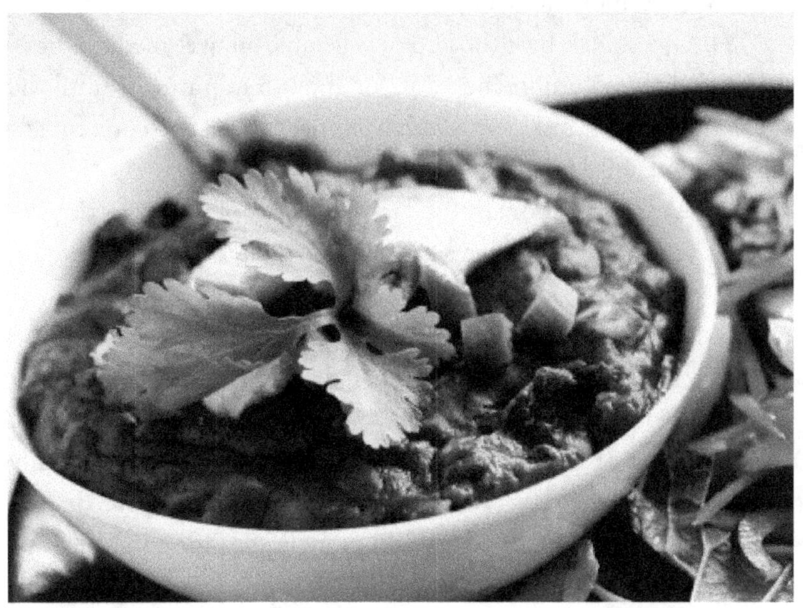

1. RINSE AND SOAK THE Beans

Start by rinsing the dried pinto beans under cold water, picking out any broken beans or debris. Soak the beans in a large bowl of water for at least 4 hours or overnight. Soaking helps soften the beans, reduces cooking time, and makes them easier to digest.

Tip: If you're short on time, you can skip soaking, but the beans will need a longer cooking time.

2. Cook the Beans

Drain the soaked beans and place them in a large pot with 6 cups of fresh water. Bring the pot to a boil, then reduce the heat to low, cover, and let the beans simmer for about 1.5 to 2 hours, or until the beans are tender. Stir occasionally and add more water if needed to keep the beans covered as they cook.

Once the beans are cooked, season them with salt to taste, but be sure to do this after they're tender; salting beans too early can make them tough.

3. Sauté Onion and Garlic

In a large skillet, heat the lard or vegetable oil over medium heat. Add the chopped onion and cook for about 5 minutes, or until the onion is soft and translucent. Add the minced garlic and cook for another minute until fragrant.

Tip: Lard is traditionally used in Mexican cooking for its rich flavor, but vegetable oil or even butter can be used for a vegetarian option.

4. Mash the Beans

Once the onions and garlic are ready, add the cooked beans to the skillet with a slotted spoon, reserving the cooking liquid. Use a potato masher or the back of a spoon to mash the beans, gradually adding some of the reserved cooking liquid to achieve your desired consistency. For creamier beans, add more liquid; for a thicker consistency, use less.

Stir the beans over medium heat for another 5-10 minutes until they reach a smooth and creamy texture. Season with additional salt if needed.

5. Serve and Garnish

Your authentic frijoles refritos are ready to serve! Spoon them into a serving dish and garnish with crumbled queso fresco and fresh cilantro if desired. Serve warm as a side dish or as a base for various Mexican dishes.

Tips for Perfect Frijoles Refritos

Use Fresh Beans: Fresher dried beans cook faster and yield a creamier texture. If your beans are older, they may take longer to cook.

Control the Consistency: For smoother beans, mash them thoroughly and add more of the cooking liquid. If you prefer a chunkier texture, leave some of the beans whole or mash them less.

Enhance Flavor with Lard: While vegetable oil works well, lard gives frijoles refritos an authentic depth of flavor. If you're using oil, a dash of smoked paprika or cumin can add a hint of smokiness.

Keep Leftover Bean Broth: The bean cooking liquid is packed with flavor and nutrients, so save any extra broth. It can be used to thin the beans as needed or added to soups and stews for additional flavor.

Variations of Frijoles Refritos

Frijoles refritos are traditionally made with pinto beans, but they can be customized to suit your taste:

Black Beans: Black beans can be used in place of pinto beans, giving the refried beans a slightly different flavor and a darker color. Black bean frijoles refritos are common in southern Mexico.

Spicy Beans: Add diced jalapeños or a pinch of cayenne pepper for a spicier version.

Cheesy Beans: Mix in shredded cheese while cooking for extra creaminess and flavor.

Serving Suggestions and Pairings

Frijoles refritos are incredibly versatile and can be served in many ways:

As a Side Dish: Serve alongside tacos, enchiladas, or grilled meats as a hearty and satisfying side.

In Burritos or Tacos: Refried beans make a great filling for burritos, tacos, and quesadillas.

As a Dip: Serve with tortilla chips and top with cheese, sour cream, and salsa for a delicious bean dip.

In Huevos Rancheros: Spread refried beans over tortillas and top with fried eggs and salsa for a classic Mexican breakfast.

The History of Frijoles Refritos

Beans have been a staple of Mexican cuisine for centuries, with frijoles refritos being one of the many ways to enjoy them. The refried cooking method highlights the versatility of beans in Mexican cooking, transforming them into a creamy, flavorful dish. Refried beans are a central part of many Mexican meals, from breakfast to dinner, and are enjoyed across Mexico and the southwestern United States.

Frequently Asked Questions

Q: Can I make frijoles refritos with canned beans?

Yes, you can use canned pinto or black beans to make refried beans if you're short on time. Simply rinse and drain the beans, then add them to the skillet with a bit of water or broth. They may need a bit more seasoning since they won't have the same depth as slow-cooked beans.

Q: How should I store leftover frijoles refritos?

Store leftover refried beans in an airtight container in the refrigerator for up to 3-4 days. They can also be frozen for up to 2 months. To reheat, add a bit of water or broth to restore the creamy consistency.

Q: Are frijoles refritos always vegetarian?

Traditionally, frijoles refritos are cooked with lard, but they can easily be made vegetarian by using vegetable oil instead. Some recipes may also include bacon or chorizo for added flavor, so be sure to check the ingredients if you're looking for a vegetarian option.

Why You'll Love This Authentic Frijoles Refritos Recipe

Frijoles refritos are comforting, creamy, and packed with flavor. This authentic recipe celebrates the simplicity and versatility of beans, transforming them into a dish that can be enjoyed in countless ways. Whether served as a side, a filling, or even a dip, frijoles refritos bring the heart of Mexican cooking to your table. With just a few ingredients and simple techniques, you can enjoy the creamy, delicious taste of homemade refried beans. Soak, simmer, and savor these classic frijoles refritos for an authentic taste of Mexican tradition.

8

Authentic Mexican Bean Soup Recipe

Mexican bean soup, or "sopa de frijol," is a traditional, heart-warming dish that's full of flavor, nutrition, and comfort. This soup combines simple ingredients—typically pinto or black beans—with Mexican spices, aromatic vegetables, and fresh toppings. The result is a rich, hearty soup that's perfect as a main course or a side. This authentic recipe keeps things simple yet delicious, allowing the beans and spices to shine.

Ingredients

1 lb. dried pinto beans or black beans (or use canned beans for a quicker version)

8 cups of water or chicken broth

1 large onion, chopped

3 garlic cloves, minced

1 jalapeño, diced (optional for heat)

2 bay leaves

1 tsp ground cumin

1/2 tsp oregano

Salt and pepper to taste

1 tbsp vegetable oil or lard

For Serving:

Freshly chopped cilantro

Lime wedges

Crumbled queso fresco or shredded cheese

Sliced avocado

Tortilla chips or warm corn tortillas

Step-by-Step Instructions

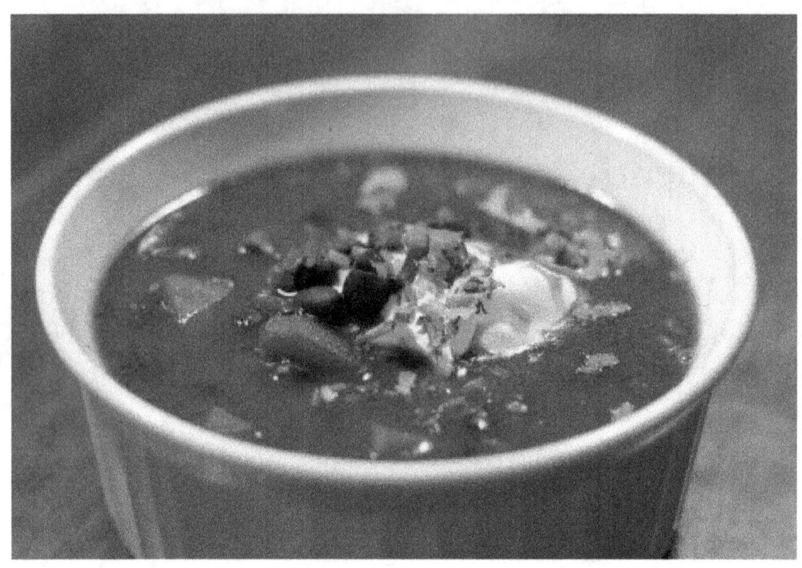

1. PREPARE THE BEANS

If you're using dried beans, start by rinsing them thoroughly and soaking them in water overnight (or for at least 6 hours). This helps reduce cooking time and makes it easier to digest. After soaking, drain and rinse the beans again.

Tip: If you're short on time, you can skip the soaking step but note that unsoaked beans will need to cook longer.

2. Cook the Beans

In a large pot, combine the soaked beans with 8 cups of water or chicken broth. Add the bay leaves, half of the chopped onion, and a pinch of salt. Bring the mixture to a boil, then reduce the heat to low, cover, and simmer for about 1.5 to 2 hours, or until the beans are tender. Stir occasionally and add more water or broth as needed to keep the beans covered.

For a quicker version, you can use canned beans; just reduce the cooking time and add less water.

3. Sauté Aromatics

In a skillet, heat the vegetable oil or lard over medium heat. Add the remaining onion, garlic, and diced jalapeño (if using). Cook for 5-7 minutes, stirring occasionally, until the onion is softened and fragrant. Add the cumin and oregano, stirring for another minute to toast the spices and enhance their flavor.

4. Combine and Simmer

Once the beans are fully cooked, add the sautéed aromatics to the pot. Stir well to combine and adjust the seasoning with salt and pepper to taste. Allow the soup to simmer for another 15-20 minutes, which lets the flavors meld together beautifully.

5. Blend for a Creamier Texture (Optional)

If you prefer a thicker, creamier soup, use an immersion blender to partially blend the soup directly in the pot. Alternatively, transfer about a third of the soup to a blender, blend until smooth, and return it to the pot. This step is optional, but it adds wonderful creaminess to the soup.

6. Serve and Garnish

Ladle the Mexican bean soup into bowls and garnish with fresh toppings like chopped cilantro, crumbled queso fresco, sliced avocado, and a squeeze of lime juice. Serve with tortilla chips or warm corn tortillas for a complete, satisfying meal.

Tips for Perfect Mexican Bean Soup

Use Fresh Ingredients: Fresh onions, garlic, and cilantro enhance the flavor of the soup and add authentic Mexican aromas.

Adjust Spice Levels: If you prefer a spicier soup, add diced jalapeño, chipotle in adobo, or a dash of cayenne. For a milder flavor, simply omit the jalapeño.

Control the Consistency: Blend part of the soup if you prefer a creamier texture, or leave it as is for a brothier consistency.

Use Homemade Broth: If possible, use homemade chicken or vegetable broth for added depth and richness. It makes a difference in the final flavor of the soup.

Variations of Mexican Bean Soup

Mexican bean soup is versatile, and there are many ways to customize it:

Add Meat: Chorizo, ham hock, or shredded chicken add heartiness and flavor to the soup. Brown the meat in the pot before adding the beans to infuse the soup with a smoky richness.

Vegetable Additions: Add diced tomatoes, zucchini, or corn to make the soup even more nutritious and colorful.

Different Beans: Black beans are commonly used, but you can try kidney beans or a mix of beans for a variety.

Serving Suggestions and Side Dishes

Mexican bean soup is a complete meal, but it also pairs well with other dishes:

Mexican Rice: Serve with Mexican rice for a fuller meal.

Cornbread or Tortillas: Warm corn tortillas, cornbread, or even crusty bread make excellent accompaniments.

Fresh Salad: A simple salad with lettuce, tomatoes, and avocado offers a refreshing contrast to the richness of the soup.

Tortilla Chips: Crumble tortilla chips on top for added crunch and flavor.

The History of Mexican Bean Soup

Beans are a staple of Mexican cuisine, with a rich history that dates back to ancient Mesoamerica, where beans were cultivated alongside corn and squash. Mexican bean soup, or "sopa de frijol," is a testament to this heritage, embodying the simplicity, nourishment, and warmth of Mexican home cooking. The dish has evolved over time, with regional variations and unique additions that reflect the diversity of Mexican culinary traditions.

Frequently Asked Questions

Q: Can I make Mexican bean soup in advance?

Yes, Mexican bean soup actually tastes even better the next day as the flavors have more time to meld. Simply store it in an airtight container in the refrigerator for up to 3-4 days. Reheat on the stove, adding a little water or broth if it's too thick.

Q: Can I freeze Mexican bean soup?

Absolutely! Mexican bean soup freezes well. Let it cool completely, then transfer it to freezer-safe containers or bags. It can be frozen for up to 3 months. To reheat, thaw in the refrigerator overnight and warm on the stove.

Q: Can I use canned beans instead of dried beans?

Yes, canned beans work well if you're short on time. Simply rinse and drain the beans, then add them to the pot with broth and aromatics. Reduce the cooking time to about 20-30 minutes, as canned beans are already tender.

Why You'll Love This Authentic Mexican Bean Soup Recipe

Mexican bean soup is a simple yet deeply satisfying dish that's easy to make, nutritious, and incredibly flavorful. The combination of tender beans, warming spices, and fresh toppings creates a bowl of comfort that's both hearty and light. This recipe captures the soul of Mexican cuisine, celebrating the flavors of traditional ingredients like beans, garlic, cumin, and lime.

Perfect for cozy nights, family dinners, or a meal-prep staple, this authentic Mexican bean soup is a versatile recipe that can be enjoyed on its own or as part of a larger spread. So grab your beans, chop those veggies, and let the aromas of Mexico fill your kitchen with this delicious, comforting soup!

9

Authentic Mexican Burrito Recipe

The burrito, a beloved Mexican dish, is a delicious combination of simple ingredients wrapped in a warm flour tortilla. Originating in the northern regions of Mexico, an authentic Mexican burrito is often smaller and focuses on a few key ingredients—usually meat, beans, and cheese. Unlike the large, overstuffed burritos commonly found in the United States, Mexican burritos are modest, letting the flavors of each component shine through. This recipe will guide you through creating an authentic, flavorful Mexican burrito with all the essentials.

Ingredients

For the Burrito Filling:

1 lb. shredded or cubed beef (such as flank steak or chuck), chicken, or pork

1 cup cooked pinto or black beans (homemade or canned, rinsed and drained)

1 cup Mexican rice (optional)

1 small onion, chopped

2 garlic cloves, minced

1 tbsp vegetable oil

1 tsp ground cumin

1 tsp chili powder

Salt and pepper to taste

For Assembly:

4-6 small flour tortillas (6-8 inches in diameter)

1/2 cup shredded Mexican cheese (queso fresco, Monterrey Jack, or cheddar)

Optional toppings: fresh salsa, guacamole, chopped cilantro

Step-by-Step Instructions

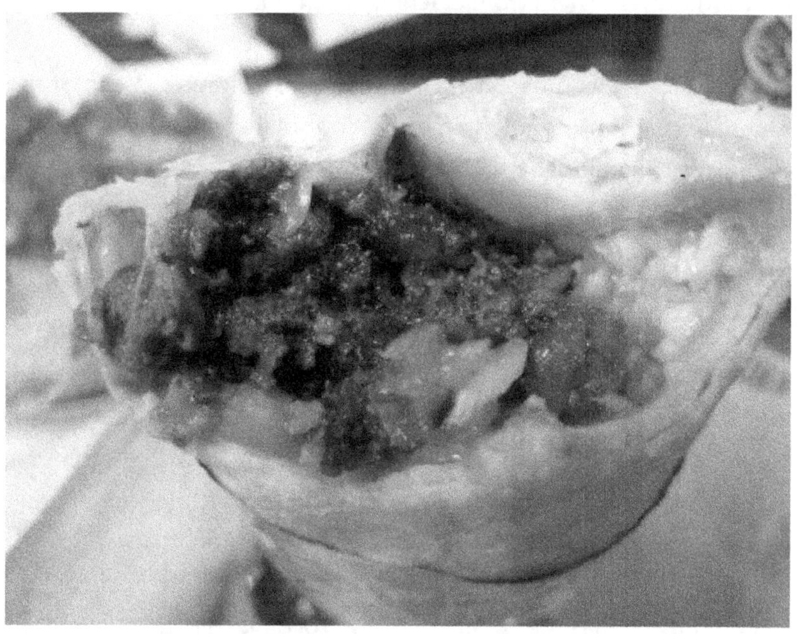

1. PREPARE THE FILLING

In a skillet, heat the vegetable oil over medium heat. Add the chopped onion and cook for about 5 minutes until it becomes soft and translucent. Add the minced garlic and cook for an additional minute until fragrant.

Add the meat to the skillet and season with cumin, chili powder, salt, and pepper. If using beef or pork, cook until the meat is tender and cooked through, about 10-15 minutes. For shredded meat, cook it until heated through and well-seasoned.

Add the cooked beans and stir well, allowing the flavors to meld for another 5 minutes. If you prefer rice in your burrito, you can add it at this stage, stirring it into the filling mixture.

2. Warm the Tortillas

Warm the flour tortillas by heating them in a dry skillet over medium heat for about 15-20 seconds on each side, or until they're soft and pliable. This step is essential to make the tortillas easier to fold and prevent them from cracking when filled.

3. Assemble the Burritos

Place a tortilla on a flat surface and spoon about 1/3 cup of the filling mixture onto the center. Sprinkle a small handful of shredded cheese over the filling.

To wrap the burrito, fold in the sides of the tortilla, then fold up the bottom and roll tightly. Repeat this process with the remaining tortillas and filling.

4. Serve and Garnish

Serve the burritos warm, with optional toppings like fresh salsa, guacamole, or chopped cilantro on the side. These toppings add freshness and flavor, but authentic Mexican burritos are often enjoyed with minimal garnishes to keep the flavors simple and focused.

Tips for Perfect Authentic Burritos

Choose the Right Tortilla: Traditional Mexican burritos use small flour tortillas. Look for soft, fresh tortillas that are easy to fold and hold the filling well.

Keep It Simple: Authentic Mexican burritos emphasize simplicity, focusing on just a few ingredients like meat, beans, and cheese. Avoid overloading with toppings, as this can detract from the authentic flavors.

Season the Filling Well: The seasoning of the meat and beans is crucial. Use fresh spices and don't be afraid to taste and adjust as you cook to get the flavor just right.

Warm the Tortillas: Heating the tortillas makes them softer and more pliable, which helps prevent them from cracking or tearing when rolled.

Variations of Mexican Burritos

While authentic burritos are simple, there are some regional variations and options you can try:

Bean and Cheese Burrito: For a vegetarian option, fill the burrito with seasoned beans and cheese for a flavorful, protein-packed meal.

Machaca Burrito: Made with shredded dried beef, this variation is popular in Northern Mexico, particularly in states like Sonora.

Chile Verde Burrito: Add a spoonful of chile verde (green chile sauce) to your burrito filling for a tangy, mildly spicy twist.

Serving Suggestions and Side Dishes

Mexican burritos are perfect on their own but can also be served with side dishes to complete the meal:

Mexican Rice: Lightly seasoned rice pairs wonderfully with burritos and makes for a satisfying meal.

Refried Beans: Creamy refried beans are a classic accompaniment and can also be added to the burrito itself.

Fresh Salsa: Serve with fresh salsa on the side for an added burst of flavor.

Guacamole: A small scoop of guacamole on the side adds creaminess and flavor.

The History of Burritos

Burritos are thought to have originated in Northern Mexico, where flour tortillas are more common due to the region's wheat cultivation. The term "burrito," meaning "little donkey" in Spanish, is said to have originated because these convenient, easy-to-carry food parcels resembled the packs that donkeys carried. Burritos have been popular in Mexican border towns and in the United States, where they evolved to include larger tortillas and more ingredients over time.

In Mexico, burritos are traditionally smaller, simpler, and often focus on a few well-seasoned ingredients. This simplicity captures the essence of authentic Mexican cooking, where each component is prepared with care and attention to flavor.

Frequently Asked Questions

Q: Can I make burritos with corn tortillas?

While corn tortillas are commonly used in Mexican cuisine, flour tortillas are traditionally used for burritos. Corn tortillas are less flexible and may crack when rolled with fillings, making flour tortillas a better choice for burritos.

Q: How can I make burritos ahead of time?

You can prepare the filling in advance and store it in the refrigerator for up to 3 days. When ready to serve, warm the filling and tortillas, assemble, and enjoy. Burritos can also be wrapped in foil and stored in the freezer for up to 2 months. Reheat in the oven or microwave.

Q: What's the difference between a burrito and a taco?

Burritos are typically made with flour tortillas and are larger, with the ingredients fully wrapped inside. Tacos are often smaller, made with corn tortillas, and usually served open-faced with fewer ingredients.

Why You'll Love This Authentic Mexican Burrito Recipe

This authentic Mexican burrito recipe captures the simplicity and flavor of traditional Mexican cuisine. With just a few high-quality ingredients, you can enjoy the rich, savory taste of seasoned meat, creamy beans, and melted cheeseball wrapped in a soft, warm tortilla. The burrito's compact size makes it perfect for a quick lunch, family dinner, or on-the-go meal. These burritos are easy to make, and their flavor is elevated by focusing on quality ingredients and simple, effective seasoning. Serve them with fresh salsa, guacamole, and your favorite Mexican sides, and enjoy a taste of Northern Mexico right in your own kitchen!

10

Authentic Mexican Chicken Enchilada Recipe

Chicken enchiladas are a staple of Mexican cuisine, celebrated for their delicious flavors and comforting appeal. Traditionally made with tender, shredded chicken, rich enchilada sauce, and soft corn tortillas, these enchiladas are baked to perfection and topped with melted cheese. This authentic recipe highlights the simple yet vibrant ingredients that make chicken enchiladas a beloved favorite in homes and restaurants across Mexico.

Ingredients

For the Chicken Filling:

2 cups cooked, shredded chicken (rotisserie chicken works great)

1 small onion, finely chopped

2 garlic cloves, minced

1 tsp ground cumin

1 tsp chili powder

Salt and pepper to taste

1/2 cup sour cream (optional, for added creaminess)

1/2 cup shredded cheese (for mixing with the chicken, optional)

For the Enchilada Sauce:

4-5 dried guajillo chiles

1-2 dried ancho chiles

2 cups of chicken broth (homemade or store-bought)

1 tbsp tomato paste

2 garlic cloves, minced

1/2 tsp ground cumin

1/2 tsp dried oregano

Salt to taste

For Assembly:

10-12 corn tortillas

1 1/2 cups of shredded cheese (such as Monterey Jack or cheddar)

Fresh cilantro, chopped, for garnish

Sliced green onions and sour cream for serving (optional)

Step-by-Step Instructions

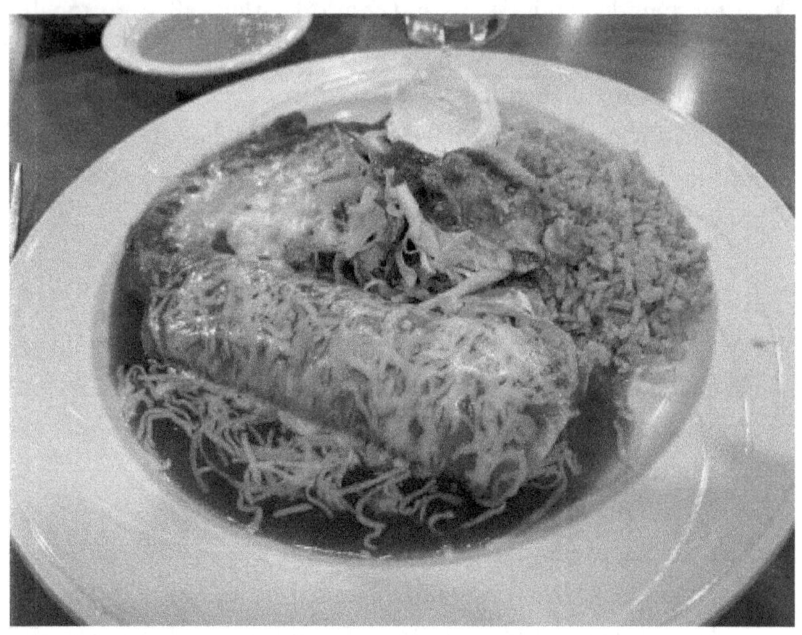

1. PREPARE THE ENCHILADA Sauce

Start by preparing the enchilada sauce. Remove the stems and seeds from the dried guajillo and ancho chiles. In a small pot, bring water to a boil, then add the chiles and let them simmer for about 5 minutes, or until they soften. Drain the chiles and place them in a blender along with chicken broth, tomato paste, minced garlic, cumin, oregano, and a pinch of salt. Blend until smooth.

In a skillet, pour the blended sauce and bring it to a simmer over medium heat. Allow it to cook for about 10-15 minutes, stirring occasionally, until the sauce thickens slightly. Adjust the seasoning as needed.

2. Prepare the Chicken Filling

In a large bowl, combine the shredded chicken, chopped onion, minced garlic, cumin, chili powder, salt, and pepper. If you want to add creaminess, mix in the sour cream and half a cup of shredded cheese. This mixture will be the flavorful filling for your enchiladas.

3. Warm the Tortillas

To make the corn tortillas pliable and prevent them from cracking, warm them in a dry skillet over medium heat for about 15-20 seconds on each side. Alternatively, you can wrap a stack of tortillas in aluminum foil and warm them in a preheated oven at 350°F (175°C) for about 10 minutes.

4. Assemble the Enchiladas

Preheat your oven to 375°F (190°C). Spread a thin layer of enchilada sauce on the bottom of a baking dish to prevent sticking.

Take a warm tortilla, spoon about 2-3 tablespoons of the chicken filling onto the center and roll it tightly. Place the rolled enchilada seam-side down in the baking dish. Repeat this process with the remaining tortillas and filling.

Once all the enchiladas are in the dish, pour the remaining enchilada sauce over the top and sprinkle with the remaining shredded cheese.

5. Bake the Enchiladas

Cover the baking dish with aluminum foil and bake in the preheated oven for about 20 minutes. Remove the foil and bake for an additional 10-15 minutes, or until the cheese is melted and bubbly.

6. Serve and Garnish

Once the enchiladas are done, remove them from the oven and let them cool for a few minutes. Garnish with fresh cilantro and sliced green onions if desired. Serve with a dollop of sour cream and your favorite sides.

Tips for Perfect Chicken Enchiladas

Use Quality Chicken: Shredded rotisserie chicken makes for an easy and flavorful filling, but you can also boil and shred your own chicken for a fresher taste.

Customize Your Sauce: Feel free to adjust the spice level of your enchilada sauce by adding a bit of cayenne pepper or fresh jalapeños if you like heat.

Don't Overfill: Be careful not to overfill the tortillas, as this can make rolling difficult and may cause the enchiladas to burst while baking.

Make Ahead: You can assemble the enchiladas ahead of time and refrigerate them until you're ready to bake. Just add a few extra minutes to the baking time if baking from cold.

Variations of Chicken Enchiladas

While the classic chicken enchilada is delicious on its own, there are many ways to customize the recipe:

Vegetarian Enchiladas: Replace the chicken with sautéed vegetables like zucchini, bell peppers, and mushrooms, and use black beans for protein.

Green Enchiladas: Substitute the red enchilada sauce with green salsa verde for a different flavor profile.

Cheesy Enchiladas: Layer extra cheese inside the enchiladas for a gooey, cheesy center.

Serving Suggestions and Side Dishes

Chicken enchiladas are delicious on their own, but they also pair well with various sides to round out the meal:

Mexican Rice: Serve with a side of Mexican rice for a hearty combination.

Refried Beans: Classic refried beans complement the enchiladas and add richness.

Guacamole and Salsa: Fresh guacamole and salsa on the side enhance the flavors and provide a refreshing contrast.

Fresh Salad: A simple salad with lettuce, tomatoes, and avocado adds freshness to the plate.

The History of Chicken Enchiladas

Enchiladas have deep roots in Mexican cuisine, tracing back to the ancient Aztecs, who would roll tortillas around small fish or other fillings. Over time, enchiladas evolved into the dish we know today, featuring a variety of fillings and sauces. The use of chicken as a filling became popular in the 20th century, reflecting the culinary preferences and ingredient availability in different regions of Mexico.

Frequently Asked Questions

Q: Can I use flour tortillas instead of corn tortillas?

While traditional enchiladas are made with corn tortillas, you can use flour tortillas if you prefer. Keep in mind that they may not have the same authentic flavor and texture, but they will still be delicious.

Q: How do I store leftovers?

Leftover chicken enchiladas can be stored in an airtight container in the refrigerator for up to 3 days. To reheat, place them in the oven at 350°F (175°C) until heated through.

Q: Can I freeze chicken enchiladas?

Yes, you can freeze enchiladas. Assemble them without baking, cover tightly, and freeze for up to 3 months. When ready to eat, bake from frozen, adding extra time to the baking process.

Why You'll Love This Authentic Mexican Chicken Enchilada Recipe

This authentic chicken enchilada recipe is a delightful blend of flavors and textures, offering a comforting meal that's perfect for any occasion. With tender shredded chicken, rich enchilada sauce, and gooey cheese, these enchiladas are a delicious expression of Mexican culinary tradition. Whether you're preparing them for a family dinner, a gathering of friends, or a cozy night in, these chicken enchiladas are sure to impress. Serve them with your favorite toppings and sides for a complete meal that showcases the heart and soul of Mexican cuisine. Enjoy the warmth and richness of this classic dish in your own kitchen!

11

Authentic Mexican Chicken Quesadilla Recipe

Chicken quesadillas are a staple of Mexican cuisine, offering a delightful blend of tender chicken, melted cheese, and soft tortillas that come together in minutes. Authentic Mexican quesadillas are typically simpler than their American counterparts, focusing on fresh ingredients and allowing the flavors of the chicken, cheese, and tortilla to shine. This recipe captures the essence of a true Mexican quesadilla, with simple seasonings and the option to add traditional fillings like fresh salsa and creamy guacamole.

Ingredients

For the Chicken Filling:

1 lb. boneless, skinless chicken breasts or thighs, cut into small strips or shredded

1 small onion, finely chopped

1 garlic clove, minced

1 tbsp vegetable oil or lard

1 tsp ground cumin

1 tsp chili powder

Salt and pepper to taste

Juice of 1 lime (optional, for added flavor)

For the Quesadilla:

8 small corn or flour tortillas (6-8 inches in diameter)

1 1/2 cups shredded Mexican cheese blend (such as queso Oaxaca, Monterey Jack, or a blend of cheeses)

Fresh cilantro, chopped (optional)

Butter or oil for cooking

Optional Toppings and Fillings:

Pico de gallo

Guacamole

Sour cream

Fresh salsa or hot sauce

Step-by-Step Instructions

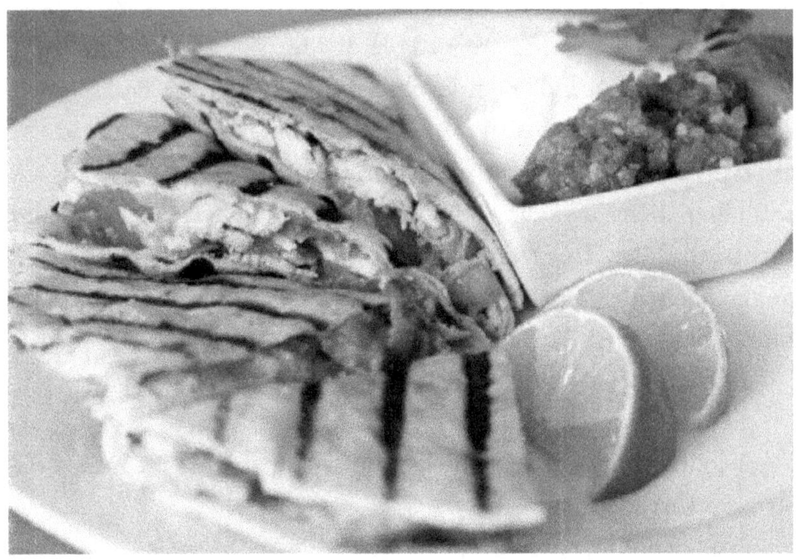

1. PREPARE THE CHICKEN

In a skillet, heat the vegetable oil or lard over medium heat. Add the chopped onion and cook for about 5 minutes, until softened. Add the minced garlic and cook for another minute until fragrant.

Add the chicken strips to the skillet and season with cumin, chili powder, salt, and pepper. Cook the chicken for 7-10 minutes, or until it is fully cooked and nicely browned. If desired, squeeze the lime juice over the chicken for extra flavor. Once cooked, set the chicken aside.

Tip: For an even simpler version, you can use leftover cooked or rotisserie chicken. Just shred it and season it with the spices before adding it to the quesadilla.

2. Assemble the Quesadilla

Heat a separate skillet or griddle over medium heat. Add a small amount of butter or oil to the pan to prevent sticking and enhance the flavor.

Place one tortilla in the skillet. Sprinkle a layer of shredded cheese over half of the tortilla, then add a few spoonsful of the cooked chicken on top. Sprinkle with a bit more cheese and, if desired, some fresh cilantro for added flavor. Fold the tortilla in half over the filling to create a half-moon shape.

3. Cook the Quesadilla

Cook the quesadilla for 2-3 minutes on each side, or until the tortilla is golden and crispy and the cheese has fully melted. Press down lightly with a spatula to help the cheese bind the quesadilla together. Once cooked, remove it from the skillet and repeat with the remaining tortillas and filling.

4. Serve and Garnish

Slice the quesadillas into wedges and serve immediately. Garnish with fresh toppings like Pico de gallo, guacamole, sour cream, and salsa for an extra burst of flavor. These toppings add a refreshing contrast to the warm, cheesy quesadilla.

Tips for Perfect Chicken Quesadillas

Use Fresh Cheese: Authentic quesadillas often use Mexican cheeses like queso Oaxaca, which melts beautifully. Monterey Jack or a Mexican cheese blend also works well for a creamy texture.

Adjust Seasonings: If you like spicier quesadillas, add a pinch of cayenne pepper or a few slices of jalapeño to the chicken filling.

Use Corn Tortillas for Authenticity: Corn tortillas add an authentic taste and texture, but flour tortillas are also widely used and can hold more filling.

Cook Slowly: Cook the quesadilla on medium heat to allow the cheese to melt evenly without burning the tortilla.

Variations of Chicken Quesadillas

While simple cheese and chicken quesadilla is classic, there are a few ways to customize your quesadilla:

Add Vegetables: Sautéed bell peppers, onions, or mushrooms make great additions for a veggie-packed quesadilla.

Go Spicy: Add sliced jalapeños or a sprinkle of hot sauce to the filling for a bit of heat.

Herb and Cheese Mix: Sprinkle fresh herbs like cilantro or a bit of Mexican oregano into the cheese for extra flavor.

Serving Suggestions and Side Dishes

Chicken quesadillas are perfect as a main dish or as a snack. Serve them with traditional Mexican sides for a complete meal:

Mexican Rice: Lightly seasoned rice is a great side dish for quesadillas.

Refried Beans: Creamy refried beans pair wonderfully with quesadillas and add extra protein.

Tortilla Soup: A small bowl of tortilla soup is a delicious starter to serve alongside quesadillas.

Simple Green Salad: A crisp green salad with avocado and tomatoes provides freshness and balance.

The History of Quesadillas

Quesadillas have roots in Mexican cuisine, where they were traditionally made with fresh corn tortillas and filled with cheese, beans, or simple ingredients like squash blossoms. As they spread across regions, various fillings like meats and vegetables became popular. In northern Mexico, flour tortillas are commonly used for quesadillas, especially in areas where wheat is cultivated. The dish's versatility and simplicity have made it popular worldwide, with countless regional variations.

Frequently Asked Questions

Q: Can I make quesadillas in advance?

Yes, you can prepare and assemble the quesadillas in advance, then cook them when ready to serve. To reheat, place them in a skillet or oven until warmed through and crispy.

Q: Can I bake quesadillas instead of cooking them on the stove?

Yes, for a hands-off approach, you can bake quesadillas in the oven. Preheat the oven to 400°F (200°C), place assembled quesadillas on a baking sheet, and bake for 8-10 minutes, flipping halfway through.

Q: Can I use store-bought rotisserie chicken?

Absolutely! Using rotisserie chicken is a convenient option. Just shred it and season it with the spices before adding it to the quesadilla.

Why You'll Love This Authentic Mexican Chicken Quesadilla Recipe

This authentic chicken quesadilla recipe is all about simplicity and flavor. The tender, seasoned chicken, melty cheese, and warm tortilla make for a comforting dish that's quick to prepare yet incredibly satisfying. Each bite captures the essence of Mexican cooking, where fresh ingredients and balanced flavors create a deliciously rich and filling meal. Perfect for family dinners, casual gatherings, or even a quick lunch, these quesadillas are versatile and crowd-pleasing. Pair them with fresh salsa, guacamole, and a squeeze of lime for a meal that will transport you to the heart of Mexican cuisine. Enjoy the classic flavors and easy preparation of this authentic Mexican chicken quesadilla recipe!

12

Authentic Mexican Red Chili Sauce Recipe

Mexican red chili sauce, also known as "salsa roja" or "chile rojo," is a versatile sauce that adds depth and boldness to countless Mexican dishes. Made with dried chiles, garlic, onions, and spices, this sauce has a smoky, slightly spicy flavor that's perfect for enchiladas, tamales, chilaquiles, and more. This authentic recipe focuses on using simple, traditional ingredients that allow the rich, earthy flavors of the chiles to shine.

Ingredients

4-5 dried guajillo chiles

2-3 dried ancho chiles

1 dried pasilla chile (optional, for added depth)

2 cups chicken or vegetable broth (or water)

1 small white onion, chopped

3 garlic cloves, peeled

1 tsp ground cumin

1/2 tsp dried oregano (Mexican oregano if available)

1/4 tsp ground cinnamon (optional, for a hint of warmth)

Salt and pepper to taste

1 tbsp vegetable oil or lard

Step-by-Step Instructions

1. Prepare the Chiles

Begin by removing the stems and seeds from the guajillo, ancho, and pasilla chiles. To intensify their flavor, toast the chiles in a dry skillet over medium heat for about 30 seconds on each side, until they're fragrant but not burnt. Toasting the chiles releases their oils and enhances the smokiness of the sauce.

2. Soak the Chiles

After toasting, transfer the chiles to a bowl and cover them with hot water. Let them soak for about 15 minutes, or until they become soft and pliable. This step makes it easier to blend the chiles into a smooth sauce.

3. Sauté the Aromatics

In a skillet, heat the vegetable oil or lard over medium heat. Add the chopped onion and cook for about 5 minutes, or until softened and translucent. Add the garlic and cook for another minute until fragrant. This will add a delicious base flavor to the sauce.

4. Blend the Sauce

Drain the softened chiles and place them in a blender along with the sautéed onions and garlic. Add the cumin, oregano, cinnamon (if using), and about 1 cup of chicken or vegetable broth. Blend until smooth, adding more broth as needed to reach your desired consistency. The sauce should be thick but pourable.

Tip: If you prefer a very smooth sauce, strain it through a fine-mesh sieve to remove any small pieces of chile skin.

5. Simmer and Season

Pour the blended sauce back into the skillet and bring it to a gentle simmer over medium-low heat. Season with salt and pepper to taste. Let the sauce simmer for about 10-15 minutes, stirring occasionally, until it thickens slightly and the flavors meld together.

Tips for Perfect Red Chili Sauce

Choose Quality Chiles: Guajillo, ancho, and pasilla chiles give this sauce a rich, complex flavor. Look for dried chiles that are soft and pliable, as older, brittle chiles can have a dull flavor.

Adjust Spice Levels: This sauce is mild to moderately spicy. If you like more heat, add a few dried arbol chiles or a pinch of cayenne pepper.

Control the Consistency: For a thicker sauce, use less broth; for a thinner, more pourable sauce, add more liquid. The sauce should be smooth but thick enough to coat the back of a spoon.

Variations of Mexican Red Chili Sauce

Mexican red chili sauce is adaptable, and there are a few ways to customize it based on your taste or the dish you're preparing:

Add Tomatoes: For a slightly sweeter, tangier sauce, add one or two roasted tomatoes to the blender.

Spicy Variation: Add a couple of dried arbol chiles for extra heat.

Roasted Vegetables: Roasting the onions and garlic before blending can add a deeper, smoky flavor to the sauce.

Serving Suggestions and Dish Pairings

This authentic Mexican red chili sauce is a versatile addition to any meal. Here are some traditional ways to enjoy it:

Enchiladas: Use the sauce as a base for authentic enchiladas rojas by dipping the tortillas in the sauce before filling and rolling them.

Tamales: Drizzle the sauce over tamales, or use it as a base for the masa to add flavor.

Chilaquiles: Pour the sauce over tortilla chips and top with cheese, sour cream, and fried eggs for a flavorful chilaquiles dish.

Tacos and Burritos: Use as a topping for tacos, burritos, or as a dip for tortilla chips.

Mexican Rice: Stir a few spoonsful into Mexican rice for added color and flavor.

The Cultural Significance of Mexican Red Chili Sauce

In Mexican cuisine, red chili sauce holds a special place as a staple ingredient. Traditional sauces made from dried chiles have been used for centuries in Mexican cooking, symbolizing the depth and complexity of regional flavors. Each region has its own version, reflecting the ingredients and culinary heritage of the area. This red chili sauce is versatile and can be adapted to different dishes, from street food to holiday feasts, making it a foundational recipe in Mexican cooking.

Frequently Asked Questions

Q: Can I make this sauce ahead of time?

Yes, you can prepare this sauce in advance and store it in the refrigerator for up to one week. It also freezes well for up to three months. Just reheat before using and adjust the consistency with a bit of water or broth if it has thickened.

Q: How spicy is this sauce?

This sauce is mildly spicy with a smoky, earthy flavor. Guajillo and ancho chiles are relatively mild, while pasilla adds a touch of depth. For a spicier sauce, add a few dried arbol chiles.

Q: Can I use this sauce as a marinade?

Absolutely! This red chili sauce makes an excellent marinade for chicken, beef, or pork. Simply coat the meat in the sauce and let it marinate for at least 30 minutes before grilling or roasting.

Why You'll Love This Authentic Mexican Red Chili Sauce Recipe

This authentic Mexican red chili sauce captures the rich, smoky, and slightly spicy flavors that elevate Mexican cuisine. With a blend of dried chiles, garlic, and spices, this sauce is both versatile and full of character. It's easy to make, and once you taste it, you'll find yourself reaching for it to enhance your favorite Mexican dishes. Whether you're making enchiladas, tamales, or simply adding a little spice to your meal, this red chili sauce is sure to become a staple in your kitchen. Embrace the traditional flavors of Mexico and bring a taste of authentic Mexican cooking to your table with this delicious sauce. Enjoy!

13

Authentic Mexican Pork Chop Recipes

Mexican cuisine offers a variety of flavorful ways to prepare pork chops, using spices, marinades, and cooking methods that bring out the natural flavors of the meat. Mexican pork chop recipes often feature ingredients like chiles, garlic, citrus, and herbs, creating dishes that are rich, savory, and full of character. Here are two classic approaches to making authentic Mexican pork chops: grilled pork chops marinated in adobo sauce, and smothered pork chops in a tangy tomatillo salsa verde.

Recipe 1: Grilled Pork Chops in Adobo Marinade

Ingredients

4 bone-in pork chops, about 1-inch thick

3 dried guajillo chiles, stemmed and seeded

2 dried ancho chiles, stemmed and seeded

1/4 cup orange juice

2 tbsp apple cider vinegar

3 garlic cloves

1 tsp ground cumin

1 tsp dried oregano (Mexican oregano if available)

Salt and pepper to taste

Fresh lime wedges for serving

Step-by-Step Instructions

1. Prepare the Adobo Marinade

Toast the dried guajillo and ancho chiles in a dry skillet over medium heat for about 30 seconds on each side, until they become fragrant. Transfer them to a bowl and cover with hot water, allowing them to soak for 10-15 minutes, until softened.

Drain the chiles and place them in a blender with orange juice, apple cider vinegar, garlic, cumin, oregano, salt, and pepper. Blend until smooth, adding a bit of water if needed to reach a thick, pourable consistency.

2. Marinate the Pork Chops

Place the pork chops in a large dish or resealable plastic bag and pour the adobo marinade over them. Make sure each chop is well coated. Cover and refrigerate for at least 1 hour, or up to overnight, for the best flavor.

3. Grill the Pork Chops

Preheat your grill to medium-high heat. Remove the pork chops from the marinade, shaking off any excess. Grill the pork chops for about 4-5 minutes per side, or until they reach an internal temperature of 145°F (63°C) and have a nice char.

4. Serve and Garnish

Serve the grilled pork chops hot, garnished with fresh lime wedges for an extra burst of flavor. These adobo-marinated pork chops are delicious served with Mexican rice, grilled vegetables, or a simple green salad.

Recipe 2: Pork Chops in Tomatillo Salsa Verde

Ingredients

4 bone-in pork chops, about 1-inch thick

Salt and pepper to taste

1 tbsp vegetable oil or lard

8-10 tomatillos, husked and rinsed

1 jalapeño or serrano pepper (optional, for heat)

1 small white onion, chopped

2 garlic cloves

1/2 cup fresh cilantro, chopped

Fresh lime wedges for serving

Step-by-Step Instructions

1. Season and Sear the Pork Chops

Season the pork-chop generously with salt and pepper. In a large skillet, heat the vegetable oil or lard over medium-high heat. Add the pork chops and sear them for about 3-4 minutes per side, until they are browned. Remove them from the skillet and set aside.

2. Prepare the Tomatillo Salsa Verde

In the same skillet, add the tomatillos, chopped onion, garlic, and jalapeño or serrano pepper if you'd like some heat. Sauté for about 5 minutes, stirring occasionally, until the tomatillos soften and begin to release their juices.

Transfer the sautéed tomatillo mixture to a blender along with fresh cilantro and a pinch of salt. Blend until smooth, adjusting seasoning as needed.

3. Simmer the Pork Chops in Salsa Verde

Return the pork chops to the skillet and pour the tomatillo salsa verde over them. Cover and simmer over low heat for about 15-20 minutes, or until the pork chops are tender and fully cooked. This process allows the pork chops to absorb the tangy, slightly spicy flavors of the salsa verde.

4. Serve and Garnish

Serve the pork chops hot, smothered in salsa verde, with fresh lime wedges on the side. They pair wonderfully with refried beans, Mexican rice, or warm corn tortillas for a complete meal.

Tips for Perfect Mexican Pork Chops

Choose Bone-In Chops: Bone-in pork chops are ideal for these recipes, as they tend to be juicier and more flavorful than boneless cuts.

Marinate for Maximum Flavor: The adobo marinade benefits from at least 1 hour of marinating, but overnight is best. The acidity in the orange juice tenderizes the meat, making it juicy and flavorful.

Control the Spice Level: Adjust the number of chiles or the type of peppers in the salsa verde to control the heat level to your preference.

Use Fresh Ingredients: Fresh tomatillos, chiles, and lime juice will enhance the authenticity and flavor of these dishes.

Variations on Mexican Pork Chops

While these two recipes are classics, there are endless ways to add Mexican flavors to pork chops:

Pork Chops al Pastor: Marinate pork chops in a pineapple and adobo marinade for a sweet and tangy twist inspired by tacos al pastor.

Pork Chops in Mole Sauce: Serve pork chops smothered in rich, complex mole sauce for an indulgent, special-occasion meal.

Chipotle-Marinated Pork Chops: Use chipotle peppers in adobo sauce for a smoky, spicy marinade, perfect for grilling or pan-searing.

Serving Suggestions

Mexican pork chops are versatile and pair well with a variety of sides:

Mexican Rice: The mild, fluffy rice complements the bold flavors of the pork chops.

Refried Beans: Creamy and savory, refried beans add richness to the meal.

Grilled Vegetables: Grilled bell peppers, zucchini, and onions make a colorful, flavorful accompaniment.

Warm Corn Tortillas: Serve with warm tortillas for scooping up the sauce or making impromptu tacos.

The Cultural Significance of Mexican Pork Chops

Pork has been a popular protein in Mexican cuisine for centuries, particularly after the introduction of pigs by the Spanish. Mexican pork dishes often incorporate traditional flavors like chiles, citrus, and herbs, creating meals that highlight regional ingredients and techniques. From slow-cooked carnitas to quick-grilled pork chops, Mexican recipes celebrate pork in diverse, flavorful ways.

Frequently Asked Questions

Q: Can I make these recipes with boneless pork chops?

Yes, you can substitute boneless pork chops but be mindful of the cooking time as they tend to cook faster. To avoid overcooking, use a meat thermometer to ensure they reach an internal temperature of 145°F.

Q: How spicy is the adobo marinade?

The adobo marinade has a mild to moderate spice level, as guajillo and ancho chiles are not very hot. If you like extra heat, you can add a chile de árbol or chipotle pepper to the marinade.

Q: Can I use a store-bought salsa

14

Authentic Mexican Soups Recipes

Mexican soups are an essential part of Mexican cuisine, celebrated for their warmth, depth of flavor, and cultural significance. From hearty stews to light broths, Mexican soups often feature ingredients like chiles, corn, tomatoes, and herbs, creating a comforting and nourishing meal. Each soup is unique to the region and reflects the local ingredients and culinary traditions. Here are some beloved authentic Mexican soups you can recreate at home.

1. Pozole Rojo (Red Hominy and Pork Soup)

Pozole is one of Mexico's most famous soups, traditionally made with hominy (large corn kernels) and pork, slowly simmered with spices and chiles. Pozole Rojo, specifically, gets its beautiful red color from dried red chiles, like guajillo and ancho, which add a mild smokiness to the broth.

Ingredients:

2 lbs. pork shoulder, cut into chunks

1 large can of hominy, drained and rinsed

4 dried guajillo chiles, stemmed and seeded

2 dried ancho chiles, stemmed and seeded

1 onion, halved

4 garlic cloves

1 tsp Mexican oregano

Salt and pepper to taste

Instructions:

Bring a large pot of water to a boil, add the pork, onion, garlic, and salt, and simmer until tender (about 2 hours).

Soak the chiles in hot water for 15 minutes, then blend with a little water until smooth. Strain if desired.

Add the hominy and chile sauce to the pot and simmer for another 30 minutes.

Serve with traditional toppings like shredded cabbage, radishes, avocado, lime wedges, and fresh cilantro.

2. Caldo de Res (Beef and Vegetable Soup)

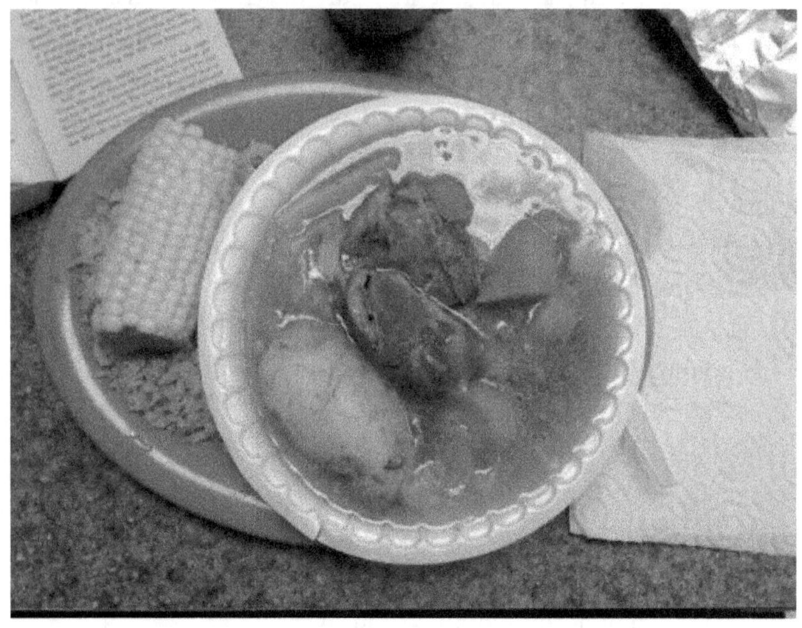

CALDO DE RES, OR MEXICAN beef and vegetable soup, is a comforting, nourishing soup made with tender beef, potatoes, carrots, cabbage, and corn. It's slow-cooked to bring out the flavors of the beef and vegetables, resulting in a rich, flavorful broth.

Ingredients:

2 lbs. beef shank or bone-in beef stew meat

2 corn ears, cut into pieces

2 carrots, chopped

1 large potato, chopped

1 zucchini, chopped

1/2 head cabbage, cut into chunks

1 onion, chopped

Salt and pepper to taste

Instructions:

In a large pot, add the beef, onion, and enough water to cover. Bring to a boil, reduce heat, and simmer until tender (about 2 hours).

Add the corn, carrots, potato, and zucchini, and simmer until the vegetables are tender.

Add the cabbage in the last 10 minutes of cooking.

Serve with lime wedges, fresh cilantro, and warm tortillas.

3. Sopa de Tortilla (Tortilla Soup)

Sopa de Tortilla is a flavorful tomato-based soup topped with crispy tortilla strips, avocado, and cheese. This light, yet comforting soup is infused with the flavors of tomatoes, chiles, and fresh herbs, making it an all-time favorite.

Ingredients:

4 tomatoes, roasted and peeled

1 onion, chopped

2 garlic cloves

4 cups of chicken broth

1-2 dried pasilla chiles, sliced

Salt to taste

Tortilla strips, avocado slices, queso fresco, and cilantro for garnish

Instructions:

Blend the roasted tomatoes with onion and garlic until smooth.

In a pot, heat oil and cook the tomato mixture for a few minutes. Add the chicken broth and simmer for 15 minutes.

Fry the pasilla chile strips in oil and set aside.

Serve the soup with fried tortilla strips, avocado, queso fresco, and fried chile strips on top.

4. Albondigas Soup (Mexican Meatball Soup)

Albondigas Soup is a hearty soup with homemade meatballs made from ground beef and rice, simmered with vegetables like potatoes, carrots, and zucchini. This soup is perfect for a comforting family meal.

Ingredients:

1 lb. ground beef

1/4 cup of uncooked rice

1 egg

2 garlic cloves, minced

1 tsp ground cumin

Salt and pepper to taste

1 onion, chopped

4 cups chicken or beef broth

2 carrots, chopped

2 potatoes, diced

1 zucchini, chopped

Fresh cilantro for garnish

Instructions:

Mix the ground beef, rice, egg, garlic, cumin, salt, and pepper. Form into small meatballs.

In a pot, sauté the onion in oil, then add the broth and bring to a simmer.

Add the meatballs and cook for 10 minutes, then add the carrots, potatoes, and zucchini. Simmer until the vegetables are tender.

Garnish with fresh cilantro and serve with warm tortillas.

5. Caldo de Pollo (Mexican Chicken Soup)

Caldo de Pollo, or Mexican chicken soup, is a simple yet deeply comforting dish. Made with chicken, vegetables, and sometimes rice, this soup is often enjoyed with fresh lime, cilantro, and warm tortillas on the side.

Ingredients:

1 whole chicken or 4 chicken legs and thighs

1 onion, quartered

2 garlic cloves

3 carrots, chopped

2 potatoes, chopped

2 zucchinis, chopped

2 corn ears, cut into pieces

Salt to taste

Instructions:

In a large pot, add the chicken, onion, garlic, and salt, then cover with water. Bring to boil, then simmer until the chicken is cooked.

Add the carrots, potatoes, zucchini, and corn, and simmer until the vegetables are tender.

Serve with lime wedges, fresh cilantro, and chopped onion.

6. Menudo (Beef Tripe Soup)

Menudo is a traditional soup made with beef tripe, hominy, and a blend of red chiles. It's often enjoyed during celebrations and is also a popular remedy for hangovers.

Ingredients:

2 lbs. beef tripe, cut into pieces

1 large can of hominy, drained and rinsed

4 dried guajillo chiles, stemmed and seeded

2 dried ancho chiles, stemmed and seeded

1 onion, chopped

2 garlic cloves

Salt to taste

Instructions:

In a large pot, add the tripe, onion, garlic, and salt, then cover with water. Simmer until the tripe is tender (about 2-3 hours).

Soak the chiles in hot water for 15 minutes, then blend with water until smooth.

Add the hominy and chile sauce to the pot and simmer for another 30 minutes.

Serve with lime wedges, chopped onion, and fresh oregano.

Tips for Making Authentic Mexican Soups

Use Fresh Ingredients: Fresh tomatoes, onions, garlic, and herbs are essential for creating a flavorful base.

Slow Cook for Rich Flavor: Mexican soups benefit from slow cooking, allowing the ingredients to fully release their flavors.

Customize with Toppings: Traditional Mexican soups are often served with garnishes like lime wedges, fresh cilantro, chopped onion, avocado, and radishes. These toppings add brightness and flavor to the finished dish.

Experiment with Chiles: Dried chiles like guajillo, ancho, and pasilla add depth and smokiness. Adjust the type and amount based on your heat preference.

Why You'll Love Authentic Mexican Soups

Authentic Mexican soups are warm, flavorful, and packed with nutrients, making them a go-to comfort food for any season. These recipes capture the heart and soul of Mexican cooking, blending simple ingredients with time-honored techniques. Whether you're making a batch of pozole for a celebration or enjoying a bowl of caldo de pollo on a cozy evening, these soups are sure to bring comfort and joy to your table. Embrace the warmth, history, and vibrant flavors of Mexican soups by trying one of these authentic recipes. Each bowl offers a taste of tradition, perfect for sharing with family and friends!

15

Authentic Pork Barbacoa Recipe

Barbacoa is a traditional Mexican dish with roots in ancient cooking methods, where meat was slow cooked in underground pits for hours until tender and infused with smoky, earthy flavors. While traditional barbacoa is often made with beef or lamb, pork barbacoa has become a beloved variation that's just as delicious. This authentic pork barbacoa recipe is seasoned with spices, chiles, and citrus, then cooked slowly to tender perfection. It's ideal for tacos, burritos, or even served on its own with classic Mexican sides.

Ingredients

4 lbs. pork shoulder or pork butt, cut into large chunks

4 dried guajillo chiles, stemmed and seeded

2 dried ancho chiles, stemmed and seeded

1 chipotle pepper in adobo sauce (for added smokiness)

1/4 cup of orange juice

1/4 cup of apple cider vinegar

1 large onion, chopped

4 garlic cloves, peeled

1 tbsp dried oregano (Mexican oregano if available)

1 tbsp ground cumin

1 tsp ground cloves

Salt and pepper to taste

2 bay leaves

1 cup chicken or beef broth

Step-by-Step Instructions

1. Prepare the Chiles

Begin by toasting the dried guajillo and ancho chiles in a dry skillet over medium heat for about 30 seconds on each side, until they become fragrant. This step helps release the oils in the chiles, enhancing their flavor. Transfer the toasted chiles to a bowl and cover them with hot water. Let them soak for about 15 minutes, or until they are softened.

2. Make the Marinade

Drain the softened chiles and place them in a blender. Add the chipotle pepper, orange juice, apple cider vinegar, chopped onion, garlic, oregano, cumin, ground cloves, salt, and pepper. Blend until smooth, adding a little water or broth if needed to create a thick, pourable paste.

3. Marinate the Pork

Place the pork chunks in a large dish or resealable plastic bag. Pour the marinade over the pork, ensuring that each piece is thoroughly coated. Cover and refrigerate for at least 2 hours, or ideally, overnight. Marinating for an extended period allows the flavors to penetrate the meat, making it even more flavorful.

4. Slow-Cook Pork

When ready to cook, preheat your oven to 275°F (135°C). Transfer the marinated pork and all the marinade into a large oven-safe pot or Dutch oven. Add the bay leaves and the broth. Cover the pot with a lid and slowly cook in the oven for 4-5 hours, or until the pork is incredibly tender and shreds easily with a fork. Alternative Cooking Methods: If you prefer, you can cook the pork barbacoa in a slow cooker on low for 8 hours or high for 5-6 hours. Alternatively, use a pressure cooker or Instant Pot and cook on high pressure for about 1 hour.

5. Shred the Pork

Once the pork is fully cooked, remove it from the oven and let it cool slightly. Use two forks to shred the pork into bite-sized pieces, mixing it with the remaining sauce in the pot to keep the meat moist and flavorful.

6. Serve and Garnish

Your pork barbacoa is ready to serve! It's perfect for tacos, burritos, or tostadas. Garnish with fresh toppings like chopped cilantro, diced onions, and a squeeze of lime juice. For a traditional Mexican touch, serve it with warm corn tortillas, rice, and beans.

Tips for Perfect Pork Barbacoa

Choose the Right Cut of Pork: Pork shoulder or pork butt is ideal for barbacoa because it's well-marbled and becomes tender when slow-cooked. Avoid lean cuts, as they can dry out during the cooking process.

Marinate for Maximum Flavor: Allowing the pork to marinate for several hours (or overnight) helps the flavors penetrate the meat, resulting in a more robust taste.

Adjust the Spice Level: The chipotle pepper adds smokiness and mild heat, but you can add another chipotle or a few arbol chiles if you like it spicier.

Save the Cooking Liquid: The rich cooking liquid is full of flavor, so mix some of it back into the shredded pork to keep it juicy and flavorful.

Variations of Pork Barbacoa

While this recipe is classic, there are a few variations you can try to customize the flavor:

Add Pineapple: Pineapple juice or chunks can be added to the marinade for a slightly sweeter, tangy flavor.

Beer Braise: Swap out some of the broth for a dark Mexican beer, which adds depth and a slight bitterness that balances the richness of the pork.

Smoky Chipotle Barbacoa: Add more chipotle peppers or even a teaspoon of smoked paprika to the marinade for an extra smoky kick.

Serving Suggestions and Side Dishes

Pork barbacoa is versatile and pairs well with many traditional Mexican sides:

Mexican Rice: The mild, fluffy rice complements the bold flavors of the barbacoa.

Refried Beans: Creamy refried beans add richness and balance to the meal.

Tortillas: Serve with warm corn or flour tortillas for wrapping the barbacoa or making tacos.

Pico de Gallo: The fresh, zesty flavor of pico de gallo pairs perfectly with the tender pork.

Guacamole: Creamy guacamole adds freshness and balances the spiciness of the barbacoa.

The History of Barbacoa

Barbacoa is a cooking tradition that dates to the indigenous peoples of the Caribbean and Mexico. Traditionally, meat was slowly cooked in underground pits lined with leaves, which infused it with a unique smoky flavor. Over time, barbacoa techniques evolved, with each region developing its own version. In northern and central Mexico, barbacoa is often made with beef, lamb, or goat. Pork barbacoa is a delicious variation that has gained popularity due to its tenderness and flavor.

Today, barbacoa is enjoyed across Mexico and the United States, often as a weekend or celebratory dish, where it's shared among family and friends. Its rich, smoky flavor and tender texture make it a beloved classic in Mexican cuisine.

Frequently Asked Questions

Q: Can I make pork barbacoa in advance?

Yes, pork barbacoa tastes even better the next day as the flavors meld. Store it in an airtight container in the refrigerator for up to 3 days. Reheat gently on the stove, adding a little broth if it needs moisture.

Q: How spicy is this pork barbacoa recipe?

This recipe is mildly spicy due to the guajillo, ancho, and chipotle chiles. You can adjust the spice level by adding more chipotles or arbol chiles for extra heat or reduce the chiles for a milder taste.

Q: Can I freeze pork barbacoa?

Yes, pork barbacoa freezes well. Store it in freezer-safe containers for up to 3 months. To reheat, thaw in the refrigerator overnight and warm on the stove with a little extra broth.

Why You'll Love This Authentic Pork Barbacoa Recipe

This authentic pork barbacoa recipe captures the essence of Mexican flavors with its smoky, tangy, and mildly spicy taste. The slow-cooked pork becomes tender and juicy, making it perfect for tacos, burritos, or simply enjoyed with rice and beans. The homemade marinade adds depth, while the slow-cooking process allows all the spices to meld beautifully. Pork barbacoa is a versatile, crowd-pleasing dish that's easy to make and brings the bold, traditional flavors of Mexico to your table. Whether you're hosting a family dinner, a casual gathering, or simply craving authentic Mexican food, this pork barbacoa will become a favorite go-to recipe. Enjoy the rich flavors and textures of this classic Mexican dish!

16

Authentic Taco Salad Recipe

Taco salad is a popular dish that brings together the bold flavors of Mexican cuisine in a light, fresh, and filling way. Unlike the versions often seen in American restaurants, which can be heavy with sour cream and cheese, an authentic Mexican taco salad emphasizes fresh ingredients like crisp lettuce, seasoned meat, beans, fresh salsa, avocado, and lime. This recipe combines all the essentials for a vibrant taco salad that's both delicious and easy to prepare.

Ingredients

For the Salad:

1 lb. ground beef, chicken, or pork (or cooked, shredded beef or chicken)

1 tbsp vegetable oil

1 tsp ground cumin

1 tsp chili powder

Salt and pepper to taste

4 cups chopped romaine or iceberg lettuce

1 cup cherry tomatoes, halved

1 cup black beans or pinto beans, rinsed and drained

1 cup corn kernels (canned, fresh, or frozen and thawed)

1 avocado, diced

1/4 cup chopped red onion

1/2 cup shredded Mexican cheese blend (optional)

Fresh cilantro, chopped, for garnish

For the Dressing:

1/4 cup fresh lime juice (about 2-3 limes)

1/4 cup olive oil

1 garlic clove, minced

1/2 tsp ground cumin

Salt and pepper to taste

For Serving:

Tortilla strips or chips for crunch

Fresh salsa or pico de gallo

Sour cream or Mexican crema (optional)

Step-by-Step Instructions

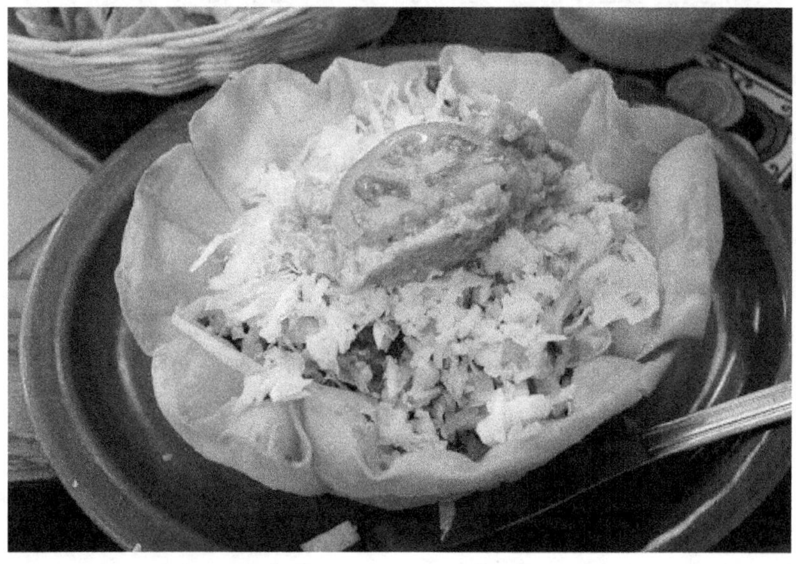

1. COOK THE MEAT

In a skillet, heat the vegetable oil over medium heat. Add the ground meat, break it up with a spoon, and cook until it begins to brown. Add the cumin, chili powder, salt, and pepper, and continue cooking until the meat is fully browned and cooked through. Taste and adjust the seasoning as needed. Set the cooked meat aside to cool slightly.

Tip: If you use shredded chicken or beef, you can skip browning and simply toss the cooked meat with the spices to flavor it.

2. Make the Lime Dressing

In a small bowl, whisk together the lime juice, olive oil, minced garlic, ground cumin, salt, and pepper. Taste and adjust seasoning if necessary. This zesty dressing complements the flavors of the salad and adds a refreshing tang.

3. Prepare the Salad Base

In a large salad bowl, add the chopped lettuce as the base. Arrange the cherry tomatoes, black beans, corn, diced avocado, and chopped red onion on top of the lettuce. Sprinkle with shredded cheese if desired.

4. Add Meat and Dressing

Add the cooked, seasoned meat to the salad. Drizzle the lime dressing over the top and toss the salad gently to coat all the ingredients evenly with the dressing.

5. Garnish and Serve

Top the salad with fresh cilantro, tortilla strips or chips, and a dollop of fresh salsa or pico de gallo. For a creamy touch, add a spoonful of sour cream or Mexican crema. Serve immediately and enjoy!

Tips for Perfect Taco Salad

Use Fresh Ingredients: Crisp lettuce, ripe tomatoes, and fresh lime juice are essential for a vibrant taco salad.

Adjust for Heat: If you like a spicier salad, add diced jalapeños or a dash of hot sauce to the dressing.

Toss Right Before Serving: To keep the lettuce and toppings crisp, toss the salad with the dressing just before serving.

Customize the Protein: Taco salad is flexible, ground beef, shredded chicken, or even grilled shrimp for variety.

Variations on Taco Salad

While the classic taco salad is delicious as is, there are plenty of ways to customize it to suit your tastes:

Vegetarian Taco Salad: Skip the meat and use additional black beans or pinto beans as the main protein. Add grilled peppers or zucchini for more flavor.

Fish Taco Salad: Swap the meat for grilled fish, such as tilapia or cod, seasoned with Mexican spices. This variation is light, refreshing, and perfect for summer.

Creamy Avocado Dressing: Blend avocado with lime juice, cilantro, and Greek yogurt or sour cream for a creamy, avocado-based dressing.

Serving Suggestions and Sides

An authentic Mexican taco salad is a meal on its own, but you can add some traditional sides to enhance the experience:

Elote (Mexican Street Corn): Grilled corn on the cob topped with mayo, cheese, and spices is a tasty side for taco salad.

Refried Beans: Serve a side of warm refried beans to complement the fresh, cool salad.

Chips and Salsa: Classic tortilla chips and salsa or guacamole are perfect for scooping up extra salad ingredients.

The Origins of Taco Salad

The taco salad is often associated with Tex-Mex cuisine rather than traditional Mexican cuisine. However, it draws inspiration from classic Mexican ingredients like beans, seasoned meat, lettuce, and fresh toppings. Over the years, taco salad has become popular across the United States and Mexico as a lighter, yet flavorful, alternative to tacos. Authentic versions of taco salad focus on fresh ingredients, simplicity, and the flavors of traditional Mexican spices.

Frequently Asked Questions

Q: Can I make taco salad ahead of time?

Yes, you can prepare most of the ingredients in advance. Keep the lettuce and fresh toppings separate from the dressing to prevent sogginess. When ready to serve, add the dressing and toss the salad.

Q: Is taco salad healthy?

Taco salad can be a nutritious meal, especially when made with fresh vegetables, lean protein, and light dressing. Opt for minimal cheese and sour cream if you're looking for a lighter option.

Q: Can I use store-bought dressing?

Yes, a good-quality store-bought dressing can be used if you're short on time. Look for a dressing with lime or cilantro for an authentic Mexican flavor.

Why You'll Love This Authentic Taco Salad Recipe

This authentic taco salad recipe is fresh, flavorful, and a satisfying twist on traditional Mexican flavors. It combines crisp lettuce, zesty lime dressing, savory seasoned meat, and classic toppings like beans, avocado, and tortilla strips, making it a crowd-pleaser that's perfect for lunch, dinner, or even a gathering. With its vibrant colors and bold flavors, taco salad is not only delicious but also visually appealing, offering a balanced meal that's packed with nutrients. Whether you're a fan of traditional tacos or looking for a lighter way to enjoy Mexican cuisine, this authentic taco salad brings the best of both worlds. It's easy to make, highly customizable, and full of the flavors and textures that make Mexican food so beloved. Enjoy a taste of Mexico with this delicious, easy-to-prepare taco salad!

17

Banana Leaf Tamales Recipe

Banana leaf tamales are a delicious variation of traditional Mexican tamales, especially popular in southern Mexico, Central America, and the Yucatán Peninsula. Unlike corn husk tamales, these are wrapped in banana leaves, which impart a unique earthy aroma and keep the masa (dough) moist and tender. The filling options are endless, but banana leaf tamales are often made with savory ingredients like pork, chicken, or vegetables, all enhanced by the flavors of fresh herbs and spices.

This recipe will guide you through making banana leaf tamales from scratch, filling them with a savory pork or chicken filling and wrapping them in banana leaves for an authentic and flavorful experience.

Ingredients

For the Masa:

3 cups masa harina (corn flour for tamales)

1 cup pork lard or vegetable shortening

2 1/2 cups chicken or pork broth (adjust as needed for consistency)

1 tsp baking powder

1 tsp of salt

For the Filling (Pork or Chicken in Red Chile Sauce):

1 1/2 lbs. pork shoulder or chicken thighs, cooked and shredded

4 dried guajillo chiles, stemmed and seeded

2 dried ancho chiles, stemmed and seeded

2 cups of chicken or pork broth

1 onion, chopped

2 garlic cloves

1 tsp ground cumin

Salt and pepper to taste

For Wrapping:

15-20 banana leaves, cut into 12-inch squares

Kitchen twine or strips of banana leaves for tying

For Serving:

Fresh salsa, lime wedges, and chopped cilantro

Step-by-Step Instructions

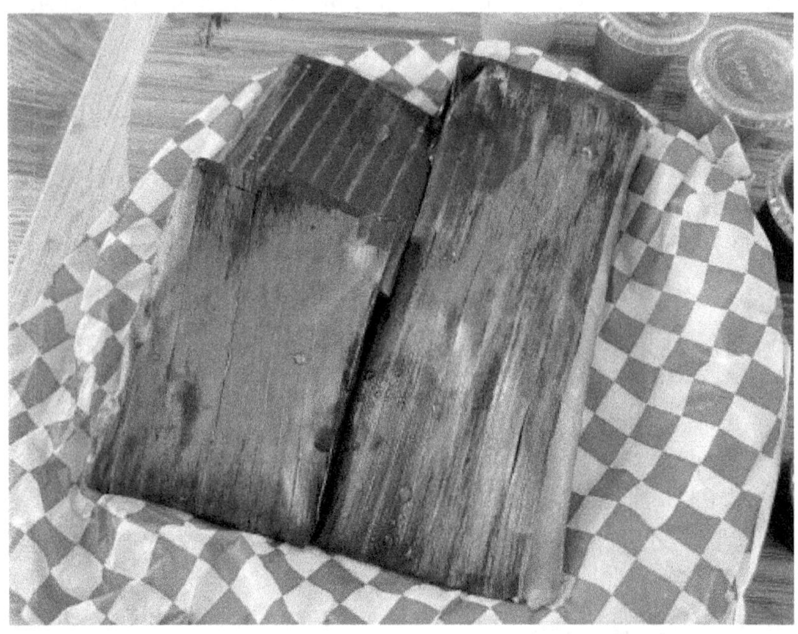

1. PREPARE THE BANANA Leaves

Banana leaves often need to be softened before they're flexible enough for wrapping. Rinse each leaf and pat it dry. Carefully pass the leaves over an open flame or place them on a hot skillet for a few seconds on each side. This will make the leaves pliable and bring out their natural aroma. Cut the leaves into squares, approximately 12 inches on each side, and set them aside.

2. Make the Filling

Soak the dried guajillo and ancho chiles in hot water for about 15 minutes, or until softened. Drain the chiles and transfer them to a blender, along with the broth, onion, garlic, cumin, salt, and pepper. Blend until smooth.

In a skillet, heat a bit of oil and pour in the chile sauce. Let it simmer for about 10 minutes, stirring occasionally, until it thickens slightly. Add the shredded pork or chicken to the sauce, stirring to coat the meat evenly. Simmer for an additional 5 minutes, then set the filling aside to cool.

3. Prepare the Masa

In a large mixing bowl, beat the lard or shortening with an electric mixer until light and fluffy. In a separate bowl, mix the masa harina, baking powder, and salt. Gradually add the masa mixture to the lard, alternating with the broth, while continuing to beat until the masa is smooth and spreadable. The masa should be fluffy but not too wet; it should hold its shape when spread on the banana leaf.

To test for readiness, drop a small ball of masa into a glass of water. If it floats, it's ready. If it sinks, beat the masa a bit longer to incorporate more air.

4. Assemble the Tamales

Place a banana leaf square on a flat surface, with the smoother side facing up. Spread about 1/4 cup of masa onto the center of the leaf, forming a rectangle about 3 inches wide. Place a spoonful of the filling in the center of the masa.

Fold the sides of the banana leaf over the filling, then fold the top and bottom to form a rectangular package. Secure the tamale with kitchen twine or by tying it with a thin strip of banana leaf.

Repeat this process with the remaining banana leaves, masa, and filling.

5. Steam the Tamales

In a large steamer pot, add water to just below the steamer basket. Line the basket with a few bananas leaves to prevent sticking. Place the tamales upright in the steamer, making sure they're packed snugly to prevent them from opening.

Cover the tamales with additional banana leaves or a damp cloth, then cover with the pot lid. Steam over medium heat for about 1.5 to 2 hours, or until the masa is firm and pulls away easily from the banana leaf.

Tip: Check the water level periodically and add more hot water as needed to keep the steam going.

6. Serve and Enjoy

Once the tamales are done, let them cool slightly. Serve the tamales in their banana leaf wrappers, allowing diners to unwrap their own. Serve with fresh salsa, lime wedges, and chopped cilantro for garnish. The banana leaf imparts a subtle, earthy flavor to the tamales, making each bite uniquely delicious.

Tips for Perfect Banana Leaf Tamales

Soften the Leaves: Passing the banana leaves overheat makes them more flexible and less likely to crack when wrapping.

Choose the Right Filling: Banana leaf tamales work well with flavorful, saucy fillings like spiced pork, chicken, or vegetarian fillings with peppers and cheese.

Pack the Tamales Well: Ensure the tamales are packed snugly in the steamer to keep them intact during steaming.

Keep Masa Light: Beating the masa with lard or shortening makes it light and fluffy, which is key for tender tamales.

Variations of Banana Leaf Tamales

Banana leaf tamales are versatile and can be made with different fillings and masa flavors:

Vegetarian Tamales: Use a filling of roasted poblano peppers, cheese, and salsa for a vegetarian option.

Sweet Tamales: For a sweet variation, add a bit of sugar to the masa and fill with a sweet filling like pineapple or chocolate.

Spicy Tamales: Add a few chile de árbol or chipotle peppers to the filling for a spicy kick.

Serving Suggestions and Side Dishes

Tamales are often served with a variety of sides that complement their rich flavors:

Mexican Rice: A side of fluffy Mexican rice pairs wonderfully with tamales.

Refried Beans: Creamy refried beans are a traditional accompaniment that adds heartiness to the meal.

Fresh Salsa: A zesty, fresh salsa brings balance to the richness of the tamales.

Guacamole: Creamy guacamole adds freshness and pairs well with tamales' savory flavors.

The Cultural Significance of Banana Leaf Tamales

Tamales have been a part of Mexican and Central American cuisine for thousands of years, dating back to the time of the Aztecs and Mayans. Banana leaf tamales are especially common in southern Mexico, where banana trees grow abundantly. The banana leaves not only impart a unique flavor but also provide a natural, eco-friendly wrapper.

Banana leaf tamales are often made for special occasions, holidays, and celebrations, where families come together to prepare large batches. Making tamales is a time-honored tradition that's passed down through generations, reflecting the importance of food, family, and community in Mexican culture.

Frequently Asked Questions

Q: Can I make banana leaf tamales in advance?

Yes, you can assemble the tamales in advance and store them in the refrigerator for up to 2 days before steaming. You can also freeze the assembled tamales and steam them directly from frozen, adding an extra 30 minutes to the steaming time.

Q: How do I reheat banana leaf tamales?

The best way to reheat tamales is by steaming them for about 10-15 minutes. You can also microwave them by wrapping them in a damp paper towel, though the texture may differ slightly.

Q: Can I use store-bought banana leaves?

Yes, store-bought frozen banana leaves work well. Thaw them and follow the same process of passing them overheated to soften them.

Why You'll Love This Authentic Banana Leaf Tamales Recipe

This authentic banana leaf tamales recipe brings a traditional Mexican flavor to your table, with tender, flavorful masa and a richly seasoned filling, all wrapped in the unique aroma of banana leaves. These tamales are a celebration of Mexican culture and cuisine, perfect for sharing with family and friends. Whether you're making them for a special occasion or simply enjoying the process of creating a beloved Mexican dish, banana leaf tamales are an experience in both taste and tradition. With their earthy aroma, tender texture, and vibrant flavors, these tamales offer a true taste of Mexico, bringing joy to anyone who unwraps them. Enjoy this authentic recipe and the delicious flavors of banana leaf tamales!

18

Beef and Bean Enchilada Recipe

Beef and bean enchiladas are a delicious and comforting Mexican dish that combines seasoned ground beef, creamy beans, and melted cheese all wrapped in soft tortillas and smothered in a flavorful red enchilada sauce. Perfect for family dinners, gatherings, or even meal prep, this recipe is simple to make and packed with flavor. Serve these enchiladas with fresh toppings like sour cream, avocado, and cilantro for a meal everyone will love.

Ingredients

For the Filling:

1 lb. ground beef

1 cup cooked pinto beans or black beans, rinsed and drained

1 small onion, finely chopped

2 garlic cloves, minced

1 tsp ground cumin

1 tsp chili powder

Salt and pepper to taste

For the Enchilada Sauce:

4 dried guajillo chiles, stemmed and seeded

1-2 dried ancho chiles, stemmed and seeded

2 cups of chicken or vegetable broth

1 tbsp tomato paste

2 garlic cloves, minced

1/2 tsp ground cumin

1/2 tsp dried oregano

Salt to taste

For Assembly:

10-12 corn or flour tortillas

1 1/2 cups shredded cheese (cheddar, Monterey Jack, or Mexican cheese blend)

Fresh cilantro, chopped, for garnish

Sliced green onions and sour cream for topping (optional)

Step-by-Step Instructions

1. Make the Enchilada Sauce

Start by preparing the enchilada sauce. Remove the stems and seeds from the guajillo and ancho chiles. In a small pot, bring water to a boil, then add the chiles and let them simmer for about 5 minutes, or until they soften. Drain the chiles and place them in a blender with chicken broth, tomato paste, minced garlic, cumin, oregano, and a pinch of salt. Blend until smooth.

In a skillet, heat a bit of oil and pour in the blended sauce. Simmer over medium heat for about 10 minutes, stirring occasionally, until the sauce thickens slightly. Adjust seasoning as needed.

2. Prepare the Beef and Bean Filling

In a large skillet, cook the ground beef over medium heat until it begins to brown, breaking it up with a spoon. Add the chopped onion and cook until softened, for about 5 minutes. Add minced garlic, cumin, chili powder, salt, and pepper, stirring well.

Once the beef is fully cooked and the onions are soft, stir in the beans. Let the mixture cook for another 2-3 minutes to combine the flavors. Set aside to cool slightly.

3. Warm the Tortillas

Warming the tortillas makes them more pliable and less likely to break when rolling. You can heat them in a dry skillet over medium heat for about 15-20 seconds on each side or wrap them in foil and warm them in the oven at 350°F (175°C) for about 10 minutes.

4. Assemble the Enchiladas

Preheat your oven to 375°F (190°C). Spread a thin layer of enchilada sauce in the bottom of a baking dish to prevent sticking.

Take a warm tortilla, spoon about 2-3 tablespoons of the beef and bean filling onto the center, and sprinkle with a little shredded cheese. Roll the tortilla tightly around the filling and place it seam-side down in the baking dish. Repeat with the remaining tortillas and filling.

Once all the enchiladas are assembled, pour the remaining enchilada sauce evenly over the top, making sure all the tortillas are well coated. Sprinkle the remaining shredded cheese on top.

5. Bake the Enchiladas

Cover the baking dish with aluminum foil and bake it in the preheated oven for about 20 minutes. Remove the foil and bake for an additional 10-15 minutes, or until the cheese is melted and bubbly.

6. Serve and Garnish

Once the enchiladas are done, remove them from the oven and let them cool slightly. Garnish with fresh cilantro, sliced green onions, and a dollop of sour cream if desired. Serve hot and enjoy yourself with your favorite sides.

Tips for Perfect Beef and Bean Enchiladas

Use Quality Tortillas: Corn tortillas are traditional, but you can also use flour tortillas for a softer texture. Warm them before filling them to make them more pliable.

Adjust the Spice Level: Add extra chili powder or a few slices of jalapeño to the beef mixture for a spicier kick.

Don't Overfill: Be careful not to overfill the tortillas, as this can make them difficult to roll and may cause them to burst.

Customize Your Toppings: Fresh toppings like chopped cilantro, green onions, and sour cream add color and flavor to the dish.

Variations of Beef and Bean Enchiladas

While this recipe is classic, there are plenty of ways to customize your enchiladas:

Vegetarian Enchiladas: Skip the beef and use extra beans and vegetables, such as sautéed peppers, onions, and zucchini, for a hearty vegetarian version.

Chicken Enchiladas: Substitute the ground beef with shredded chicken for a lighter but equally delicious option.

Cheesy Enchiladas: For extra cheesiness, add a layer of cheese inside each enchilada as well as on top.

Serving Suggestions and Side Dishes

Beef and bean enchiladas pair wonderfully with traditional Mexican sides:

Mexican Rice: Serve with a side of fluffy Mexican rice for a filling and complete meal.

Refried Beans: Creamy refried beans add richness and complement the enchiladas.

Fresh Salad: A crisp green salad with lettuce, tomatoes, and avocado provides a refreshing contrast to the rich flavors of the enchiladas.

Chips and Guacamole: Serve with a side of chips and guacamole for a satisfying appetizer.

The History of Enchiladas

Enchiladas are a traditional Mexican dish that dates to ancient times, with origins in Aztec and Mayan cultures. The dish was originally made by wrapping food in corn tortillas, often accompanied by chiles and spices. Enchiladas have evolved over time, with each region of Mexico adding its own twist, creating countless variations with different sauces, fillings, and toppings. Beef and bean enchiladas are a popular adaptation that combines classic Mexican flavors with protein-rich ingredients.

Frequently Asked Questions

Q: Can I make enchiladas ahead of time?

Yes, you can assemble the enchiladas in the baking dish, cover them, and refrigerate for up to a day before baking. Add the sauce just before baking to keep the tortillas from getting too soft.

Q: How do I reheat enchiladas?

Reheat enchiladas in the oven at 350°F (175°C) for about 10-15 minutes until warmed through. You can also microwave them, though the texture may be slightly softer.

Q: Can I freeze beef and bean enchiladas?

Yes, enchiladas freeze well. Wrap them tightly in the foil and freeze for up to 3 months. To reheat, bake directly from frozen at 350°F (175°C) for about 30-40 minutes, or until heated through.

Why You'll Love This Beef and Bean Enchilada Recipe

This beef and bean enchilada recipe is a satisfying, crowd-pleasing meal that brings the flavors of Mexico right to your table. The combination of seasoned beef, creamy beans, melted cheese, and rich enchilada sauce makes each bite comforting and flavorful. These enchiladas are easy to customize, making them perfect for family dinners, potlucks, or any gathering. Serve them with your favorite Mexican sides, garnish with fresh toppings, and enjoy a taste of traditional Mexican cuisine with this delicious beef and bean enchilada recipe!

19

Beef Chimichanga Recipe

Achimichanga is essentially a deep-fried burrito, filled with deliciously seasoned beef, beans, cheese, and sometimes rice. Originating in the Southwest United States and inspired by Mexican cooking, beef chimichangas have become a beloved Tex-Mex classic, with a crispy exterior and a savory, satisfying filling. This recipe will guide you through making the perfect beef chimichanga at home, with a golden, crunchy shell and a rich, flavorful filling that's perfect for topping with fresh salsa, guacamole, and sour cream.

Ingredients

For the Beef Filling:

1 lb. ground beef or shredded beef (such as cooked chuck roast)

1 small onion, finely chopped

2 garlic cloves, minced

1 tsp ground cumin

1 tsp chili powder

1/2 tsp smoked paprika (optional, for added flavor)

Salt and pepper to taste

1/2 cup of refried beans (optional, for added creaminess)

1/2 cup shredded Mexican cheese blend (cheddar or Monterey Jack)

1/4 cup cooked rice (optional)

For the Chimichangas:

6 large flour tortillas

Vegetable or canola oil for frying

Toothpicks (to secure the chimichangas)

For Topping:

Fresh salsa or pico de gallo

Sour cream or Mexican crema

Guacamole

Chopped fresh cilantro

Step-by-Step Instructions

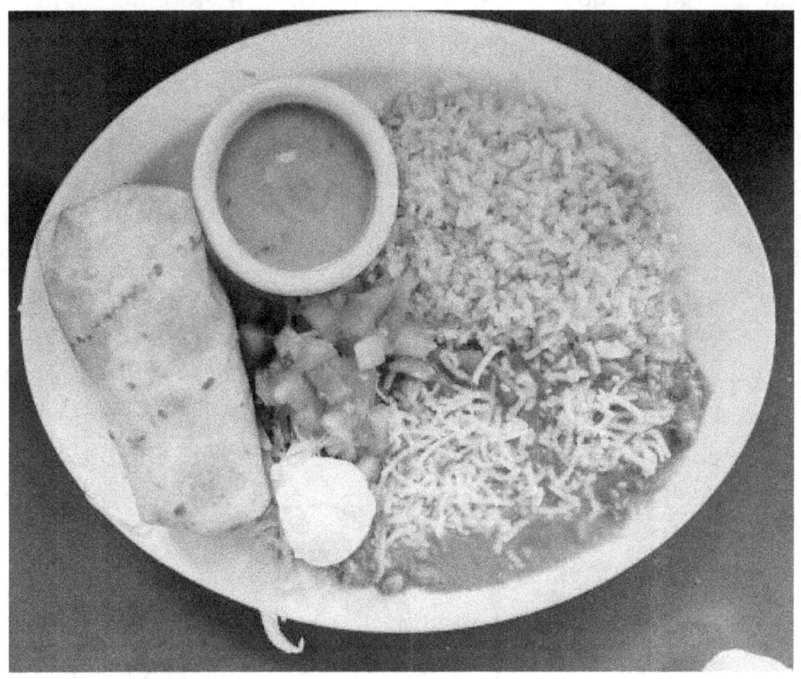

1. PREPARE THE BEEF Filling

In a large skillet over medium heat, cook the ground beef until browned, breaking it up as it cooks. Add the chopped onion and cook for about 5 minutes, or until softened. Add the minced garlic, cumin, chili powder, smoked paprika, salt, and pepper, stirring well to coat the beef in the spices.

If you're using shredded beef, simply heat it through and mix with the spices and onions. Stir in the refried beans and rice (if using) and let the mixture simmer for a few minutes, allowing the flavors to meld. Remove from heat and let the filling cool slightly before assembling the chimichangas.

2. Assemble the Chimichangas

Lay a flour tortilla on a clean, flat surface. Spoon a generous amount of the beef filling into the center of the tortilla. Top with a sprinkle of shredded cheese. Fold in the sides of the tortilla, then fold the bottom up and roll it tightly, securing it with a toothpick if necessary to prevent it from unrolling while frying.

Repeat this process with the remaining tortillas and filling.

3. Fry the Chimichangas

In a deep skillet or pot, heat about 1 inch of oil over medium-high heat until it reaches 350°F (175°C). If you don't have a thermometer, you can test the oil by dropping a small piece of tortilla in; if it sizzles and bubbles, the oil is ready.

Carefully place one or two chimichangas in the hot oil, seam-side down. Fry for about 2-3 minutes per side, or until golden brown and crispy. Use tongs to turn them as needed to ensure even frying on all sides. Once they're golden and crispy, transfer them to a paper towel-lined plate to drain excess oil. Repeat with the remaining chimichangas.

Alternative Baking Option: For a lighter option, you can brush the assembled chimichangas with a bit of oil and bake them in a preheated oven at 400°F (200°C) for about 20-25 minutes, flipping halfway through, until golden and crispy.

4. Serve and Garnish

Place the crispy chimichangas on a plate and garnish with your favorite toppings. Serve with fresh salsa, guacamole, sour cream, and a sprinkle of fresh cilantro. Enjoy your homemade chimichangas while they're hot and crispy!

Tips for Perfect Beef Chimichangas

Use Large Tortillas: Large flour tortillas are best for wrapping and can hold plenty of filling without tearing.

Secure the Tortilla: Use a toothpick to keep the tortilla tightly wrapped while frying to prevent it from unraveling.

Adjust the Filling: Customize the filling to your preference by adding ingredients like rice, beans, or even sautéed peppers for extra flavor and texture.

Keep Oil Temperature Steady: To prevent the chimichangas from getting greasy, maintain the oil at a steady temperature. If it's too low, the chimichangas may absorb too much oil.

Variations of Beef Chimichangas

Chimichangas are versatile and can be customized in various ways:

Cheesy Chimichangas: For a gooier filling, add a layer of melted cheese inside or on top after frying.

Shredded Beef Chimichangas: Use shredded beef instead of ground beef for a heartier texture. Cook the beef in a slow cooker or pressure cooker with Mexican spices, then shred it and mix with cheese and other filling ingredients.

Vegetarian Chimichangas: Skip the beef and use a filling of beans, cheese, rice, and sautéed vegetables like bell peppers and onions.

Serving Suggestions and Side Dishes

Beef chimichangas are delicious on their own but can be served with traditional Mexican sides for a complete meal:

Mexican Rice: A side of fluffy Mexican rice is a classic accompaniment.

Refried Beans: Serve with creamy refried beans for extra heartiness.

Fresh Salad: A fresh green salad with lettuce, avocado, and tomatoes adds a refreshing contrast to the crispy chimichangas.

Chips and Salsa: Tortilla chips and salsa are a perfect starter or side to enjoy with chimichangas.

The History of Chimichangas

Chimichangas have roots in the southwestern United States, particularly in Arizona and Texas, where Mexican and American flavors come together to create unique Tex-Mex dishes. Legend has it that chimichangas were invented by accident when a burrito was dropped into a fryer. The result was so delicious that it became a popular Tex-Mex specialty, with countless variations developed over the years.

Today, chimichangas are a popular menu item in Tex-Mex and Mexican-American restaurants, offering a delightful combination of crispy tortilla and savory filling.

Frequently Asked Questions

Q: Can I make chimichangas in advance?

Yes, you can prepare the filling and assemble the chimichangas ahead of time. Store them in the refrigerator for up to 1 day before frying. If you want to freeze them, wrap each chimichanga individually in plastic wrap, then place in a freezer bag. They can be fried or baked directly from frozen, just add a few extra minutes to the cooking time.

Q: What's the difference between a burrito and a chimichanga?

The main difference is that chimichangas are fried, giving them a crispy exterior, while burritos are typically served soft and unfried. Chimichangas are also usually topped with salsa, sour cream, and other garnishes.

Q: Can I use a different meat for chimichangas?

Absolutely! Shredded chicken, pork, or even ground turkey work well as alternatives to beef. Just season them similarly to the beef in this recipe.

Why You'll Love This Beef Chimichanga Recipe

This beef chimichanga recipe is a comforting, indulgent dish with the perfect combination of textures and flavors. The crispy tortilla, seasoned beef filling, and melted cheese make each bite satisfying and delicious. The fresh toppings like salsa, guacamole, and sour cream add brightness and richness, making this dish a true crowd-pleaser.

Whether you're cooking for family, friends, or simply craving a Tex-Mex favorite, these chimichangas are easy to make and even easier to enjoy. Give this recipe a try for a delicious meal that's sure to impress!

20

Black Bean Burrito Recipe

B lack bean burritos are a delicious, protein-packed option for a quick and satisfying meal. Filled with creamy black beans, fresh vegetables, and flavorful spices, these burritos are perfect for both vegetarians and anyone looking for a lighter, healthier option. Easy to make and highly customizable, black bean burritos are great for lunch, dinner, or meal prep.

This recipe keeps things simple yet flavorful, allowing the black beans and fresh toppings to shine. Top with guacamole, salsa, and a sprinkle of cheese for a burrito that's packed with flavor and nutrients.

Ingredients

For the Black Bean Filling:

1 tbsp olive oil

1 small onion, chopped

2 garlic cloves, minced

1 tsp ground cumin

1 tsp chili powder

1/2 tsp smoked paprika (optional)

1 can (15 oz) black beans, rinsed and drained

Salt and pepper to taste

Juice of 1/2 lime

For Assembly:

4 large flour tortillas

1/2 cup of cooked rice (optional)

1/2 cup shredded cheese (cheddar or Monterey Jack)

1/2 cup chopped tomatoes or salsa

1 avocado, sliced or mashed

Fresh cilantro, chopped, for garnish

Optional Toppings:

Sour cream or Greek yogurt

Fresh salsa or pico de gallo

Shredded lettuce

Hot sauce

Step-by-Step Instructions

1. Prepare the Black Bean Filling

In a skillet, heat the olive oil over medium heat. Add the chopped onion and cook for about 5 minutes, or until softened. Add the minced garlic and cook for another minute until fragrant.

Stir in the cumin, chili powder, and smoked paprika, letting the spices toast for 30 seconds to release their flavor. Add the black beans and a splash of water (about 1/4 cup) to create a saucy texture. Season with salt and pepper to taste, then cook for 5-7 minutes, stirring occasionally. Finish by adding a squeeze of lime juice for brightness.

2. Warm the Tortillas

To make the tortillas pliable and easier to roll, heat them in a dry skillet over medium heat for about 15-20 seconds on each side. Alternatively, wrap them in foil and warm in a preheated oven at 350°F (175°C) for about 5-10 minutes.

3. Assemble the Burritos

Place a warmed tortilla on a flat surface. Spread a few spoonsful of the black bean mixture onto the center of the tortilla. Add a scoop of cooked rice, a sprinkle of cheese, chopped tomatoes or salsa, and a few slices of avocado. Top with fresh cilantro.

To roll the burrito, fold the sides of the tortilla in toward the center, then fold up the bottom and roll tightly. Repeat with the remaining tortillas and filling.

4. Serve and Enjoy

Serve the black bean burritos as they are, or top them with additional salsa, sour cream, or Greek yogurt. Add shredded lettuce for extra crunch, or drizzle with hot sauce for a spicy kick. Enjoy your burritos warm and fresh!

Tips for Perfect Black Bean Burritos

Use Fresh Ingredients: Fresh toppings like cilantro, tomatoes, and lime juice enhance the flavor of the burritos.

Customize the Filling: Add other vegetables like bell peppers, corn, or sautéed mushrooms for extra texture and flavor.

Keep the Tortillas Warm: Warm tortillas are easier to roll and help keep the burrito intact.

Add Creaminess: Mash a bit of the avocado inside the burrito or spread a layer of sour cream on the tortilla for added creaminess.

Variations of Black Bean Burritos

While this recipe is classic, there are plenty of ways to customize your black bean burritos:

Spicy Black Bean Burritos: Add diced jalapeños to the filling or a few dashes of hot sauce for extra heat.

Breakfast Black Bean Burritos: Add scrambled eggs and breakfast potatoes for a hearty breakfast version.

Cheesy Black Bean Burritos: Melt additional cheese in the filling for a gooier, creamier burrito.

Serving Suggestions and Side Dishes

Black bean burritos are filling on their own, but they can be paired with other Mexican-inspired sides for a complete meal:

Mexican Rice: Serve with a side of fluffy Mexican rice for added flavor.

Refried Beans: Creamy refried beans make a hearty side to complement the black bean burrito.

Tortilla Chips and Salsa: Enjoy with a side of tortilla chips and fresh salsa or guacamole.

Corn Salad: A fresh corn and avocado salad add color and flavor to the meal.

The Origins of Burritos

Burritos are thought to have originated in Northern Mexico, where flour tortillas are more commonly used than corn tortillas. Traditionally, Mexican burritos are smaller and simpler, often filled with just one or two ingredients like beans, meat, or cheese. Over time, burritos evolved to include more ingredients and toppings, particularly in the United States, where they became a popular Tex-Mex dish with numerous variations.

Black bean burritos are a nutritious, plant-based adaptation of the classic, offering a filling meal that's both satisfying and healthy.

Frequently Asked Questions

Q: Can I make black bean burritos ahead of time?

Yes, you can assemble the burritos ahead of time and store them in the refrigerator for up to 2 days. Wrap each burrito in foil and re-heat in the oven or microwave before serving.

Q: Can I freeze black bean burritos?

Yes, black bean burritos freeze well. Wrap each burrito in plastic wrap or foil, then store in a freezer-safe bag. To reheat, remove the plastic wrap, wrap in a damp paper towel, and microwave, or bake in the oven until warmed through.

Q: Are black bean burritos healthy?

Yes, black bean burritos are a nutritious option. Black beans are rich in protein and fiber, making these burritos filling and heart-healthy. Add fresh veggies, skip heavy cheese, and limit sour cream for a lighter meal.

Why You'll Love This Black Bean Burrito Recipe

This black bean burrito recipe is quick, easy, and filled with wholesome ingredients that make it both delicious and nutritious. The seasoned black beans are packed with flavor, and the fresh toppings add a burst of color and texture. Perfect for any meal, black bean burritos are great for on-the-go lunches, casual dinners, or meal prep.

With customizable fillings and toppings, these burritos are a crowd-pleaser that everyone can enjoy. Whether you're vegetarian or simply looking for a lighter, healthier alternative to a meat-filled burrito, this recipe is the perfect choice. Enjoy the simplicity, flavor, and versatility of homemade black bean burritos!

21

Blackened Fish Taco Recipe

Blackened fish tacos are a delicious way to enjoy tender, flaky fish seasoned with bold spices and topped with fresh, vibrant ingredients. With a crispy char on the outside and juicy flavor within, blackened fish pair perfectly with soft corn tortillas, tangy slaw, and a zesty lime crema. This recipe offers a balance of spice and freshness, making it ideal for a casual dinner or a festive gathering.

Ingredients

For the Blackened Fish:

1 lb. white fish fillets (such as tilapia, cod, or mahi-mahi)

2 tbsp olive oil

1 tbsp paprika

1 tsp ground cumin

1 tsp garlic powder

1 tsp onion powder

1/2 tsp dried oregano

1/2 tsp thyme

1/2 tsp cayenne pepper (adjust for spice level)

Salt and pepper to taste

For the Slaw:

2 cups shredded cabbage (green, purple, or a mix)

1/4 cup chopped fresh cilantro

1/4 cup sliced green onions

Juice of 1 lime

1 tbsp olive oil

Salt and pepper to taste

For Lime Crema:
1/2 cup sour cream or Greek yogurt
Juice of 1 lime
1/4 tsp garlic powder
Salt to taste
For Assembly:
8 small corn tortillas
Fresh salsa or pico de gallo (optional)
Additional lime wedges for serving
Step-by-Step Instructions

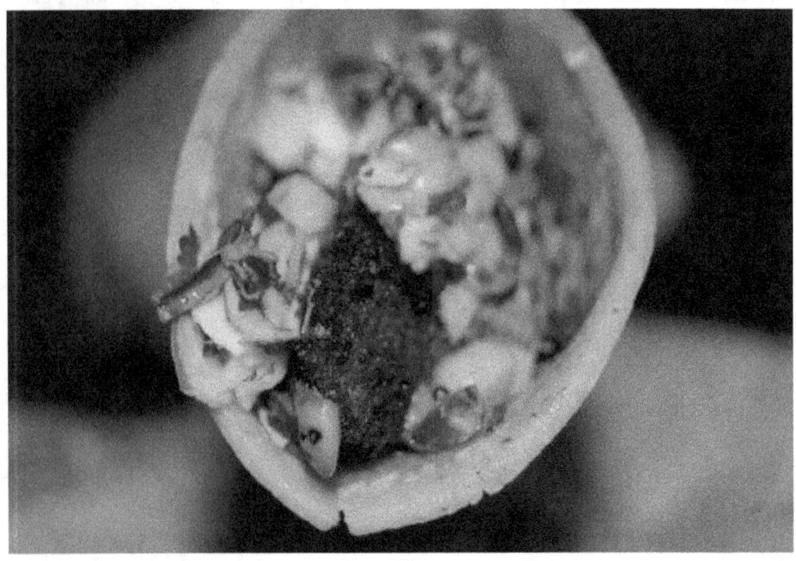

1. PREPARE THE BLACKENED Seasoning

In a small bowl, combine the paprika, cumin, garlic powder, onion powder, oregano, thyme, cayenne pepper, salt, and pepper. This mixture will be the blackened seasoning that coats the fish, giving it that signature spicy, smoky flavor.

2. Season the Fish

Pat the fish fillets dry with a paper towel, then drizzle both sides with olive oil. Rub the blackened seasoning onto both sides of each fillet, ensuring they're well coated.

3. Cook the Fish

Heat a large cast-iron skillet or nonstick pan over medium-high heat. Once hot, add a little olive oil to the pan, then place the fish fillets in the skillet. Cook for 3-4 minutes per side, or until the fish is blackened on the outside and flakes easily with a fork. The fish should have a nice, dark crust but not be burnt. Once cooked, remove the fish from the pan and set aside.

4. Prepare the Slaw

In a mixing bowl, combine the shredded cabbage, chopped cilantro, and green onions. Drizzle with lime juice and olive oil, then season with salt and pepper. Toss to combine and set aside. This slaw adds a refreshing crunch that balances the spiciness of the fish.

5. Make the Lime Crema

In a small bowl, mix the sour cream (or Greek yogurt), lime juice, garlic powder, and a pinch of salt. Stir until smooth. This tangy crema brings a cooling element to the tacos and complements the spice of the blackened fish.

6. Warm the Tortillas

Heat the corn tortillas in a dry skillet over medium heat for about 10-15 seconds per side, or until they're warm and pliable. Alternatively, you can warm them directly over a gas flame for a few seconds on each side to get a slight char.

7. Assemble the Tacos

Break the blackened fish into large chunks. Place a few pieces of fish on each tortilla, then top with a scoop of the cabbage slaw. Drizzle with the lime crema and add a spoonful of salsa or pico de gallo if desired. Garnish with extra cilantro and serve with lime wedges on the side.

Tips for Perfect Blackened Fish Tacos

Choose the Right Fish: White fish like tilapia, cod, or mahi-mahi work best for blackened fish tacos because they're mild, tender, and flaky. Thicker fillets are easier to handle in the skillet.

Adjust Spice Level: If you prefer less heat, reduce the cayenne pepper in the seasoning. For extra spice, add more cayenne or top with jalapeño slices.

Use Fresh Tortillas: Fresh corn tortillas enhance the flavor and texture of the tacos. Warming them up makes them pliable and adds flavor.

Don't Overcrowd the Pan: Cook the fish in batches if needed to avoid overcrowding, which ensures each piece gets that perfect blackened crust.

Variations of Blackened Fish Tacos

These tacos are versatile and can be customized with different ingredients and flavors:

Shrimp Tacos: Use the same blackened seasoning on shrimp instead of fish for a quick, flavorful variation.

Avocado and Mango Salsa: Add diced avocado or mango to the slaw or as a topping for a tropical twist.

Creamy Avocado Sauce: Swap out the lime crema for a creamy avocado sauce by blending avocado, lime juice, sour cream, and fresh cilantro.

Serving Suggestions and Side Dishes

Blackened fish tacos pair well with a variety of Mexican-inspired sides:

Mexican Rice: A side of fluffy Mexican rice complements the bold flavors of the tacos.

Refried Beans: Creamy refried beans add richness and balance to the meal.

Chips and Salsa: Tortilla chips with salsa, guacamole, or queso dip are great for starting the meal.

Grilled Corn Salad: A fresh corn salad with cilantro, lime, and a sprinkle of cotija cheese brings color and flavor to the table.

The Origin of Blackened Fish

Blackening as a cooking method is often associated with Cajun cuisine, particularly in Louisiana, where it was popularized by chef Paul Prudhomme in the 1980s. The technique involves coating fish (or other proteins) in a blend of spices and cooking it in a hot skillet, creating a flavorful crust. In Mexican and Tex-Mex cuisine, blackened fish has become a popular choice for tacos, offering a smoky, spicy flavor that pairs well with fresh toppings and soft tortillas.

Frequently Asked Questions

Q: Can I grill the fish instead of pan-searing it?

Yes! Grilling works well for blackened fish tacos. Simply oil the grill grates and cook the fish over medium-high heat until it's charred and flaky, about 3-4 minutes per side.

Q: What's the best way to reheat leftover fish tacos?

To keep the fish crispy, reheat it in a hot skillet for a few minutes on each side or in an oven at 350°F (175°C) for 10 minutes. Avoid microwaving, as it can make the fish rubbery.

Q: Can I use flour tortillas instead of corn tortillas?

Absolutely! While corn tortillas are traditional, flour tortillas work well if you prefer a softer, slightly thicker wrap.

Why You'll Love This Blackened Fish Taco Recipe

This blackened fish taco recipe is the perfect balance of bold spices and fresh ingredients. The blackened seasoning adds a smoky, slightly spicy crust to the tender fish, while the cabbage slaw and lime crema bring a refreshing contrast. Each bite is a satisfying blend of textures and flavors, from the crunch of the slaw to the creamy crema and tangy lime juice.

These blackened fish tacos are great for casual dinners, Taco Tuesday, or even a summer gathering with friends. Quickly preparing and bursting with flavor, they're sure to become a favorite. Enjoy the taste of fresh, homemade blackened fish tacos with this easy, authentic recipe!

174 **ADIDAS WILSON**

22

Breakfast Burrito Sauce Recipe

A great breakfast burrito isn't complete without a flavorful sauce that brings all the ingredients together. A breakfast burrito sauce should be creamy, tangy, and a little spicy, complementing the flavors of eggs, cheese, potatoes, and your choice of fillings. This versatile sauce can be drizzled inside the burrito or served on the side for dipping, adding a burst of flavor that makes every bite irresistible.

This recipe offers a quick and easy breakfast burrito sauce that combines creamy ingredients with tangy lime and a hint of spice for a balanced, satisfying taste. It's perfect not only for breakfast burritos but also as a dip for other breakfast dishes like hash browns, tacos, and more.

Ingredients

1/2 cup of mayonnaise

1/4 cup sour cream or Greek yogurt

Juice of 1 lime (about 1-2 tbsp)

1-2 tsp hot sauce (such as Cholula or Tabasco, adjust to taste)

1 tsp chipotle powder or smoked paprika (for smoky flavor)

1/2 tsp garlic powder

1/2 tsp onion powder

1/4 tsp cumin

Salt and pepper to taste

1 tbsp fresh cilantro, finely chopped (optional, for extra freshness)

Step-by-Step Instructions

1. Combine the Ingredients

In a medium bowl, combine the mayonnaise and sour cream (or Greek yogurt). Whisk until smooth and creamy. Add the lime juice, hot sauce, chipotle powder or smoked paprika, garlic powder, onion powder, and cumin. Whisk until all the ingredients are well combined.

2. Adjust Seasoning

Taste the sauce and add salt and pepper to taste. If you like extra heat, add a bit more hot sauce or a pinch of cayenne pepper. For added freshness, stir in the chopped cilantro.

3. Chill the Sauce

For best results, let the sauce chill in the refrigerator for about 10-15 minutes to allow the flavors to melt. This also helps the sauce thicken slightly, making it perfect for drizzling or dipping.

4. Serve

Your breakfast burrito sauce is ready! Drizzle it inside your breakfast burrito before rolling it up or serve it on the side for dipping. This creamy, zesty sauce also pairs well with breakfast tacos, scrambled eggs, and roasted potatoes.

Tips for Perfect Breakfast Burrito Sauce

Adjust the Heat: For a milder sauce, use less hot sauce and skip the chipotle powder. For more spice, add a little extra hot sauce, cayenne pepper, or even a few drops of sriracha.

Use Fresh Lime Juice: Fresh lime juice adds brightness and acidity, enhancing the flavor of the sauce. Avoid bottled lime juice, as it may taste less fresh.

Experiment with Yogurt: Greek yogurt can be used instead of sour cream for a slightly tangier sauce with extra creaminess.

Add Fresh Herbs: Fresh cilantro adds a bright, herbaceous note that works well in this sauce, but you can also use fresh parsley or chives for variation.

Variations of Breakfast Burrito Sauce

This sauce is versatile, and there are several ways to customize it to your taste:

Avocado Burrito Sauce: Blend the sauce with half an avocado for a creamy, avocado-based sauce with a mild green color.

Spicy Jalapeño Sauce: Blend in a few slices of fresh or pickled jalapeño for an extra kick.

Tomatillo Cream Sauce: Add a few tablespoons of blended tomatillo salsa for a tangy, green sauce that is paired beautifully with eggs and potatoes.

Serving Suggestions

While this sauce is perfect for breakfast burritos, it also pairs well with a variety of breakfast dishes:

Breakfast Tacos: Drizzle the sauce over scrambled egg tacos or breakfast quesadillas.

Hash Browns or Breakfast Potatoes: Use the sauce as a dip for crispy potatoes or hash browns.

Egg Sandwiches: Spread a little sauce on your breakfast sandwiches or bagels for added flavor.

Mexican Breakfast Bowls: Use the sauce to top a breakfast bowl with eggs, beans, rice, and avocado.

Frequently Asked Questions

Q: How long does this sauce last in the refrigerator?

This breakfast burrito sauce can be stored in an airtight container in the refrigerator for up to 3-4 days. Give it a stir before using, as it may separate slightly.

Q: Can I make this sauce dairy-free?

Yes, you can make this sauce dairy-free by using dairy-free sour cream or yogurt. You can also use a blend of mayonnaise and a squeeze of lime for a creamy, dairy-free alternative.

Q: Is there a way to make this sauce vegan?

To make this sauce vegan, substitute both the mayonnaise and sour cream with vegan alternatives. Many grocery stores offer vegan mayonnaise and sour cream, which work well in this recipe.

Q: What other seasonings can I add to this sauce?

Feel free to experiment with additional seasonings! Ground coriander, smoked paprika, or even a pinch of cayenne can add interesting flavors. Fresh herbs like chives or parsley also add brightness.

Why You'll Love This Breakfast Burrito Sauce Recipe

This breakfast burrito sauce is creamy, zesty, and easy to make with pantry staples. Its balance of creaminess, spice, and acidity complements the hearty flavors of breakfast burritos, from scrambled eggs to spicy sausage and crispy potatoes. The lime juice and fresh cilantro bring brightness to the sauce, while the chipotle powder or smoked paprika adds a hint of smokiness that elevates any breakfast dish.

Whether you're looking for a delicious sauce for breakfast burritos, a versatile dip for potatoes, or a topping for breakfast bowls, this sauce has you covered. Enjoy the flavor boost with every bite!

23

Sopas De Pollo Recipe

Sopas de pollo, or Mexican chicken soup, is a comforting, nourishing dish that's deeply rooted in Mexican cuisine. Known for its simple yet flavorful ingredients, Sopas de pollo is a popular meal for cozy family dinners and is often served when someone is feeling under the weather. This recipe combines tender chicken, fresh vegetables, and aromatic spices for a delicious, warming soup that's easy to prepare and satisfying for any occasion.

Ingredients

1 whole chicken or 4 chicken legs and thighs

10 cups of water or chicken broth

1 onion, halved

3 garlic cloves, peeled

3 carrots, peeled and chopped

2 potatoes, peeled and chopped

2 zucchinis, chopped

2 ears of corn, cut into pieces

1/2 head cabbage, chopped (optional)

1 tsp salt, or to taste

Fresh cilantro for garnish

Lime wedges for serving

Optional Toppings:

Fresh chopped cilantro

Diced avocado

Sliced jalapeño or pickled jalapeños

Warm corn tortillas

Step-by-Step Instructions

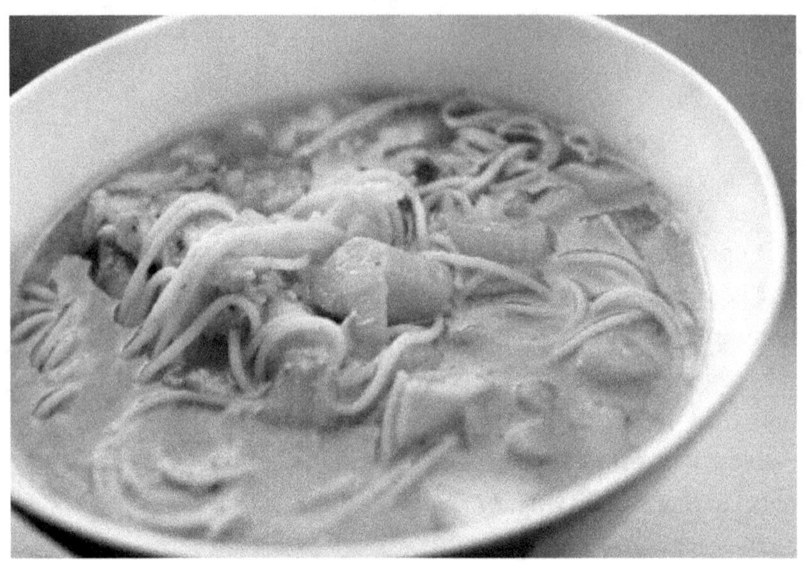

1. COOK THE CHICKEN

In a large pot, add the whole chicken (or chicken legs and thighs), water or chicken broth, onion halves, garlic cloves, and a pinch of salt. Bring the mixture to a boil, then reduce the heat to low, skimming off any foam that rises to the top. Simmer for about 30-40 minutes, or until the chicken is cooked through and tender.

2. Shred the Chicken

Once the chicken is fully cooked, remove it from the pot and let it cool slightly. Shred the chicken meat using two forks, discarding the skin and bones. Set the shredded chicken aside.

3. Add the Vegetables

In the same pot with the broth, add the chopped carrots, potatoes, zucchini, corn pieces, and cabbage if using. Season with additional salt if needed. Simmer for 15-20 minutes, or until the vegetables are tender but not overcooked.

4. Return the Chicken to the Pot

Once the vegetables are tender, add the shredded chicken back into the pot. Stir to combine and let the soup simmer for another 5 minutes to allow the flavors to meld together.

5. Serve and Garnish

Ladle the hot Sopas de pollo into bowls, making sure each bowl has a good mix of chicken, vegetables, and broth. Garnish with fresh cilantro and serve with lime wedges on the side for a burst of citrus flavor.

Serve the soup with warm corn tortillas, avocado slices, or even a side of Mexican rice for a complete, comforting meal.

Tips for Perfect Sopas de Pollo

Use Bone-In Chicken: Bone-in chicken adds richness and depth to the broth, giving the soup a more authentic flavor.

Adjust Vegetables: Sopas de pollo is versatile; add or swap vegetables based on your preference or availability. Chayote, green beans, or even spinach can be great additions.

Simmer Slowly: Cooking the soup at a gentle simmer helps keep the chicken tender and ensures a clear, flavorful broth.

Add Fresh Toppings: Fresh toppings like avocado, cilantro, and lime juice enhance the flavor of the soup and give it a refreshing finish.

Variations of Sopas de Pollo

This classic recipe can be adapted in many ways to suit your taste:

Spicy Sopas de Pollo: Add a sliced jalapeño or a dash of hot sauce to the broth for a spicier soup.

Tomato-Based Sopas de Pollo: Add a few tomatoes or a can of diced tomatoes for a richer, slightly tangy broth.

Rice and Chicken Soup: Add 1/2 cup of cooked rice to each bowl before serving for a heartier version of the soup.

Serving Suggestions and Side Dishes

While sopas de pollo is filling on its own, you can serve it with a variety of sides to create a complete meal:

Mexican Rice: A side of fluffy Mexican rice is a classic accompaniment.

Corn Tortillas: Warm corn tortillas are perfect for scooping up the broth and adding texture.

Sliced Avocado: Creamy avocado adds a cool, refreshing contrast to the hot soup.

Fresh Salsa: Serve with a side of pico de gallo or your favorite salsa for extra flavor.

The Cultural Significance of Sopas de Pollo

In Mexico, Sopas de pollo is a beloved comfort food that's often enjoyed with family. It's known for its health benefits and is commonly served to help boost immunity and provide comfort during cold seasons. Traditionally, this soup is prepared with simple, fresh ingredients, making it a wholesome meal that's suitable for all ages.

Sopas de pollo is often made in large batches, shared with loved ones, and enjoyed with plenty of warm tortillas and fresh toppings. It's a staple that's cherished for its flavor, simplicity, and nourishing qualities.

Frequently Asked Questions

Q: Can I make sopas de pollo in advance?

Yes, sopas de pollo tastes even better the next day as the flavors meld together. Store the soup in an airtight container in the refrigerator for up to 3 days. Reheat gently on the stove.

Q: Can I freeze sopas de pollo?

Yes, this soup freezes well. Store it in freezer-safe containers for up to 3 months. To reheat, thaw in the refrigerator overnight and warm on the stove.

Q: What's the best way to add more flavor to the broth?

If you'd like a richer broth, use chicken broth instead of water, or add a few extra garlic cloves, herbs, or even a squeeze of lime juice.

Q: Can I use store-bought rotisserie chicken?

Yes, rotisserie chicken can be used if you're short on time. Simply shred the cooked chicken and add it to the broth along with the vegetables, adjusting the cooking time accordingly.

Why You'll Love This Sopas de Pollo Recipe

Sopas de pollo is a comforting, nourishing, and delicious dish that's perfect for any occasion. The tender chicken, fresh vegetables, and aromatic broth make it a flavorful and healthy meal that's both easy to make and satisfying to eat. The beauty of this soup lies in its simplicity, using just a few ingredients to create a wholesome and rich meal. Whether you're feeling under the weather, craving a warm, cozy dish, or just looking for an easy family dinner, sopas de pollo is a classic recipe that brings people together. Top it with fresh cilantro, a squeeze of lime, and serve with warm tortillas for a taste of traditional Mexican comfort food. Enjoy every spoonful!

24

Soy Chorizo Recipe

Soy chorizo is a delicious plant-based alternative to traditional Mexican chorizo, made with crumbled soy and bold spices that mimic the rich, smoky flavor of pork chorizo. This vegan-friendly version is packed with spices like paprika, cumin, and garlic, offering a savory, satisfying taste without the meat. Perfect for tacos, burritos, breakfast scrambles, or even as a topping for salads, soy chorizo is versatile, easy to make, and a great way to add protein and flavor to your meals.

Ingredients

1 cup of textured vegetable protein (TVP)

1 cup vegetable broth or water

2 tbsp olive oil

1 tbsp apple cider vinegar

1 small onion, finely chopped

3 garlic cloves, minced

1 tbsp smoked paprika

1 tbsp regular paprika

1 tsp ground cumin

1 tsp ground coriander

1/2 tsp dried oregano

1/2 tsp thyme

1/2 tsp chili powder (or more, to taste)

1/4 tsp ground cloves (optional, for depth)

Salt and pepper to taste

Optional: A pinch of cayenne pepper for extra heat

Step-by-Step Instructions

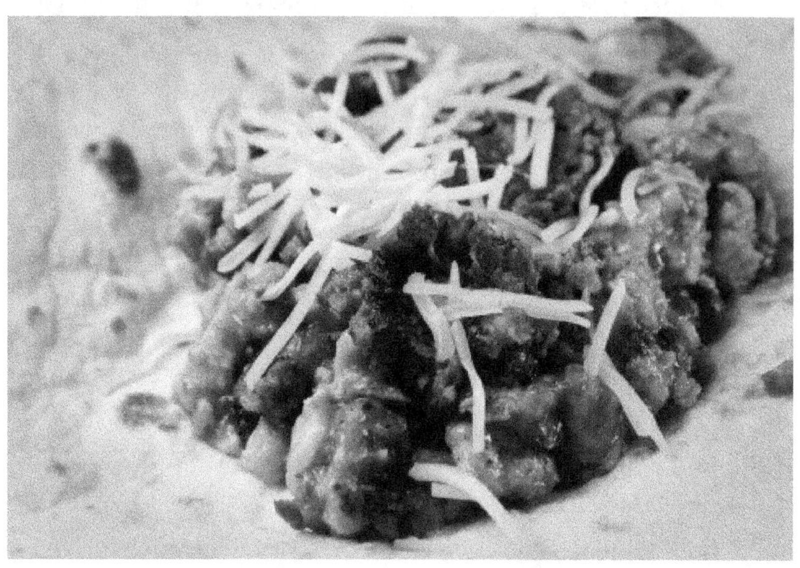

1. REHYDRATE THE TEXTURED Vegetable Protein (TVP)

In a medium bowl, add the TVP and pour the hot vegetable broth or water over it. Stir to combine and let the mixture sit for about 10 minutes, or until the TVP absorbs all the liquid and softens. Fluff with a fork once hydrated.

2. Cook the Aromatics

In a large skillet, heat the olive oil over medium heat. Add the chopped onion and cook for about 5 minutes, or until softened and translucent. Add the minced garlic and cook for another minute until fragrant.

3. Season the TVP

Once the onion and garlic are cooked, add the rehydrated TVP to the skillet. Stir well to combine the onion and garlic. Add the smoked paprika, regular paprika, cumin, coriander, oregano, thyme, chili powder, and ground cloves (if using). Mix thoroughly, coating the TVP in the spices.

4. Add Vinegar and Adjust Seasoning

Pour the apple cider vinegar into the mixture and stir. This gives the chorizo a slightly tangy taste that's characteristic of traditional chorizo. Season with salt and pepper to taste, and add a pinch of cayenne pepper if you prefer a spicier chorizo. Continue to cook for 5-7 minutes, allowing the flavors to meld.

5. Taste and Serve

Taste the soy chorizo and adjust seasoning as needed, adding more salt, spices, or vinegar if desired. Your soy chorizo is ready to serve! Use it as a filling for tacos, burritos, or as a topping for breakfast dishes like scrambled tofu or eggs.

Tips for Perfect Soy Chorizo

Choose High-Quality TVP: Textured vegetable protein (TVP) is a great base for soy chorizo, providing a texture like ground meat. You can find it in most grocery stores or health food stores.

Adjust the Spice Level: If you like a spicier chorizo, add more chili powder or a pinch of cayenne pepper. For milder chorizo, reduce or omit the cayenne.

Let It Rest: For an even more flavorful soy chorizo, let it cool and refrigerate overnight. This allows the flavors to deepen.

Use Fresh Spices: Fresh paprika, cumin, and garlic will enhance the flavor of your soy chorizo, giving it a richer taste.

Variations of Soy Chorizo

While this recipe is classic, there are several ways to customize your soy chorizo:

Chipotle Soy Chorizo: Add one or two chopped chipotle peppers in adobo sauce for a smoky, spicy twist.

Tomato-Based Chorizo: Add a few tablespoons of tomato paste for added depth and a touch of sweetness.

Mushroom and Soy Chorizo: Add finely chopped mushrooms to the TVP for a heartier texture and an earthy flavor.

Serving Suggestions

Soy chorizo is incredibly versatile and can be used in a variety of dishes:

Tacos: Spoon the soy chorizo into warm corn tortillas, top with diced onions, cilantro, and a squeeze of lime.

Breakfast Burritos: Use soy chorizo as a filling for breakfast burritos with scrambled eggs, potatoes, and cheese.

Burrito Bowls: Layer soy chorizo with rice, beans, lettuce, salsa, and avocado for a delicious burrito bowl.

Chorizo Quesadillas: Sprinkle soy chorizo with cheese inside a tortilla for a savory quesadilla.

Scrambled Tofu or Eggs: Mix the soy chorizo with scrambled tofu or eggs for a hearty, protein-packed breakfast.

The Origins of Chorizo

Chorizo has its origins in Spain and Portugal, where it's typically made from pork and seasoned with garlic and smoked paprika. When it spread to Latin America, each region created its own version, using local spices and ingredients. Mexican chorizo is generally spicier and has a red color from the addition of spices like paprika and chili powder. Soy chorizo is a modern, plant-based adaptation that captures the bold flavors of traditional chorizo while being vegan-friendly and lighter in fat.

Frequently Asked Questions

Q: Can I make soy chorizo in advance?

Yes, soy chorizo tastes even better after sitting for a few hours or overnight in the refrigerator. Store it in an airtight container for up to 5 days.

Q: Can I freeze soy chorizo?

Yes, soy chorizo freezes well. Place it in a freezer-safe container or bag, and store it for up to 3 months. Thaw it in the refrigerator before reheating in a skillet.

Q: Can I use tofu instead of TVP?

Yes, you can use crumbled firm tofu in place of TVP. Cook the crumbled tofu with the spices in a similar way to achieve a flavorful chorizo alternative.

Q: Is soy chorizo spicy?

This recipe has a mild to moderate spice level. Adjust the amount of chili powder or add cayenne pepper if you prefer a spicier flavor.

Why You'll Love This Soy Chorizo Recipe

This homemade soy chorizo recipe is full of smoky, spicy flavors that make it a delicious plant-based alternative to traditional chorizo. It's easy to prepare, versatile, and perfect for a variety of dishes, from breakfast scrambles to tacos. The combination of paprika, cumin, garlic, and vinegar gives the soy chorizo a depth of flavor that's both satisfying and full of character.

Whether you're vegan, vegetarian, or simply looking for a flavorful meat substitute, this soy chorizo recipe is a must-try. Enjoy it in tacos, burritos, or any dish that calls for chorizo, and experience the bold, delicious taste of plant-based Mexican-inspired cuisine.

25

Spinach Tortilla Recipe

Homemade spinach tortillas are a delicious and nutritious twist on classic flour tortillas. With the addition of fresh spinach, these tortillas not only gain a beautiful green color but are also packed with vitamins and minerals. They're perfect for making wraps, burritos, quesadillas, or even as a base for breakfast tacos. This easy recipe shows you how to make soft, flavorful spinach tortillas at home with just a few simple ingredients.

Ingredients

2 cups of all-purpose flour (or a mix of whole wheat and all-purpose flour)

1 cup fresh spinach leaves, packed (about 2-3 handfuls)

1/2 cup warm water (plus more as needed)

1/4 cup vegetable oil or olive oil

1/2 tsp salt

1/2 tsp baking powder

Step-by-Step Instructions

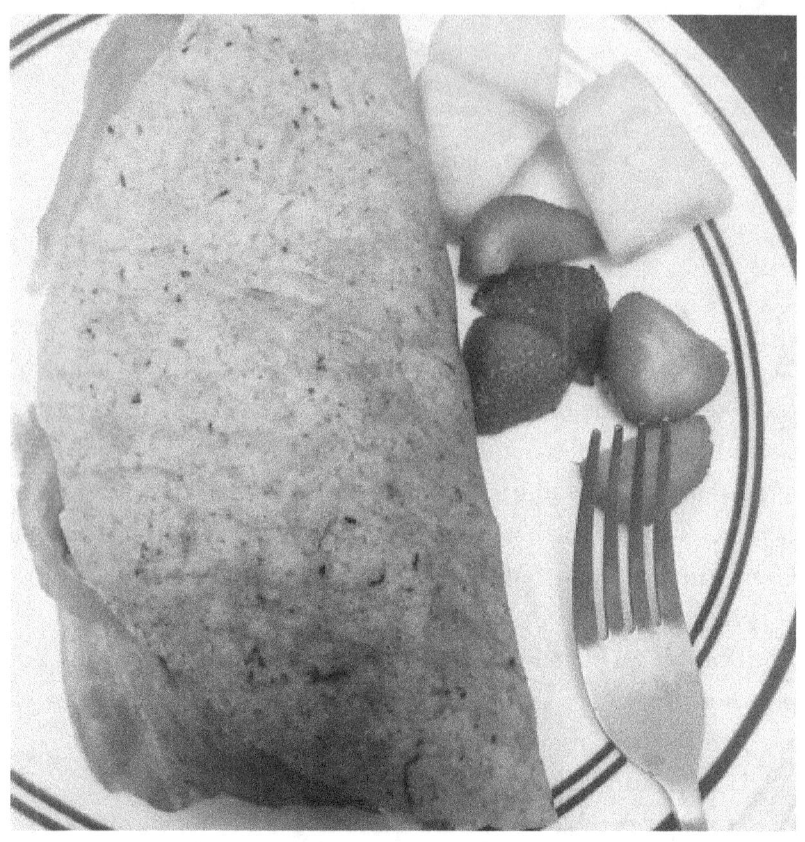

1. BLEND THE SPINACH

In a blender, combine the fresh spinach leaves with warm water. Blend until the mixture is smooth and the spinach is fully pureed. The liquid should be a vibrant green color. Set aside.

2. Prepare the Dough

In a large mixing bowl, combine the flour, salt, and baking powder. Stir to mix the dry ingredients evenly. Add the vegetable oil and the spinach mixture, stirring to combine. The dough should start to come together; if it's too dry, add a bit more water, one tablespoon at a time.

3. Knead the Dough

Turn the dough out onto a lightly floured surface. Knead the dough for about 5-7 minutes, or until it becomes smooth and elastic. If the dough is sticky, add a little more flour. Once the dough is soft and pliable, cover it with a clean kitchen towel and let it rest for 15-20 minutes. Resting allows the gluten to relax, making the tortillas easier to roll out.

4. Divide and Roll Out the Dough

After resting, divide the dough into 8-10 equal portions, depending on how large you want your tortillas. Roll each portion into a small ball. Using a rolling pin, roll each ball into a thin circle on a floured surface, about 6-8 inches in diameter. Try to keep the thickness consistent for even cooking.

5. Cook the Tortillas

Heat a large, dry skillet or griddle over medium-high heat. Once hot, place a tortilla in the skillet and cook for about 30-45 seconds, or until bubbles begin to form on the surface. Flip the tortilla and cook the other side for another 30-45 seconds, or until it has light brown spots. Remove the tortilla from the skillet and cover with a kitchen towel to keep it warm. Repeat with the remaining dough balls.

6. Serve and Enjoy

Your spinach tortillas are ready to enjoy! Serve them warm as wraps, or use them as a base for tacos, burritos, or quesadillas. Any leftover tortillas can be stored in an airtight container in the refrigerator for up to 3 days.

Tips for Perfect Spinach Tortillas

Adjust Consistency: If the dough is too sticky, add a bit more flour. If it's too dry, add a touch more water.

Blend Thoroughly: Make sure the spinach is fully blended with the water to avoid any large pieces in the dough, which could make it harder to roll out smoothly.

Rest the Dough: Allowing the dough to rest makes it easier to roll out and prevents it from shrinking back.

Use Fresh Spinach: Fresh spinach works best in this recipe, but you can also use frozen spinach. Just be sure to thaw and drain it well before blending.

Variations of Spinach Tortillas

These spinach tortillas are versatile and can be customized in different ways:

Whole Wheat Spinach Tortillas: Use half whole wheat flour and half all-purpose flour for a heartier, more nutritious tortilla.

Herbed Spinach Tortillas: Add a tablespoon of fresh herbs like basil or cilantro to the blender with the spinach for an extra layer of flavor.

Garlic Spinach Tortillas: Add a clove of garlic to the spinach when blending for a subtle garlic flavor that complements many dishes.

Serving Suggestions

Spinach tortillas can be used in many creative ways:

Wraps and Sandwiches: Use spinach tortillas as a base for wraps with fillings like hummus, grilled chicken, veggies, or turkey.

Breakfast Burritos: Fill the tortillas with scrambled eggs, cheese, and veggies for a nutritious breakfast burrito.

Quesadillas: Make spinach quesadillas with cheese, black beans, or your favorite fillings for a quick, delicious meal.

Taco Shells: Use the spinach tortillas as soft taco shells and fill them with seasoned meat, beans, or grilled veggies.

The Benefits of Spinach Tortillas

Spinach tortillas offer a nutrient boost over regular flour tortillas, thanks to the added spinach. Spinach is rich in vitamins A, C, and K, along with iron and calcium. Incorporating spinach into tortillas is a great way to increase your veggie intake, especially for picky eaters or children. Plus, the vibrant green color adds visual appeal and makes meals feel fun and healthy!

Frequently Asked Questions

Q: Can I make spinach tortillas ahead of time?

Yes! Spinach tortillas can be made in advance. Store them in an airtight container in the refrigerator for up to 3 days. Reheat them in a dry skillet or microwave before serving.

Q: Can I freeze spinach tortillas?

Absolutely. Allow the tortillas to cool completely, then stack them with parchment paper between each tortilla and place them in a freezer-safe bag. Freeze for up to 3 months. To reheat, thaw in the refrigerator and warm in a skillet.

Q: Can I make gluten-free spinach tortillas?

Yes, try using a gluten-free flour blend that's suitable for tortillas. The texture may differ slightly, so experiment with different brands to find the best result.

Q: Can I use baby spinach instead of regular spinach?

Yes, baby spinach works well and has a milder flavor than mature spinach leaves.

Why You'll Love This Spinach Tortilla Recipe

This spinach tortilla recipe is easy, wholesome, and adds a nutritious twist to traditional tortillas. The mild flavor of spinach blends well with the flour, creating a tortilla that's soft, flexible, and perfect for wraps, tacos, or burritos. The vibrant green color adds visual appeal and makes meals feel fresh and exciting.

Whether you're looking for a nutritious option for your kids' lunches, a healthy wrap base, or simply a way to incorporate more veggies, these spinach tortillas are a fantastic choice. Enjoy making these soft, green tortillas from scratch and adding a healthy boost to your favorite meals!

26

Guacamole Recipe

Guacamole is a beloved Mexican dip made from creamy avocados, fresh lime juice, and flavorful seasonings. It's simple yet delicious, making it a versatile accompaniment for tacos, burritos, nachos, or simply as a dip with tortilla chips. This classic guacamole recipe brings out the best in fresh ingredients, resulting in a deliciously rich and creamy dip with just the right balance of tang, spice, and texture.

Ingredients

3 ripe avocados

1 small onion, finely chopped

1-2 small tomatoes, finely diced (optional)

1-2 jalapeños or serrano peppers, finely chopped (remove seeds for less heat)

2 tbsp fresh cilantro, chopped

Juice of 1-2 limes (adjust to taste)

Salt to taste

Freshly ground black pepper (optional)

Optional Toppings:

Additional cilantro for garnish

A sprinkle of smoked paprika or chili powder for extra flavor

Diced mango or pineapple for a sweet twist

Step-by-Step Instructions

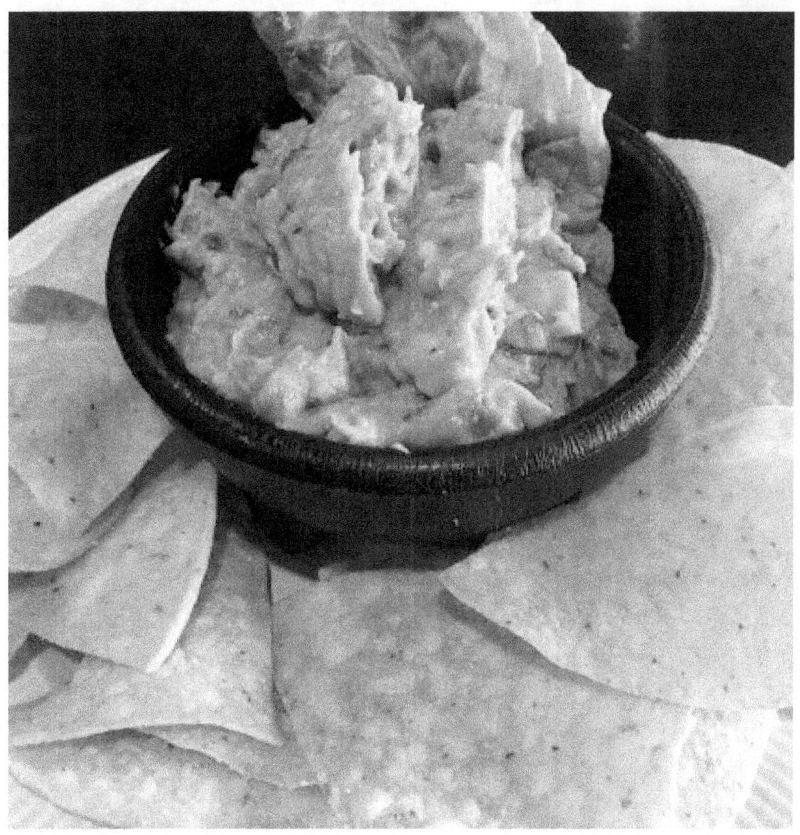

1. PREPARE THE AVOCADOS

Cut the avocados in half, remove the pits, and scoop the flesh into a mixing bowl. Choose ripe avocados that give slightly when pressed; this ensures they're soft and creamy.

2. Mash the Avocados

Using a fork or potato masher, mash the avocados to your desired texture. For a chunkier guacamole, leave some larger pieces intact. For a smoother guacamole, mash thoroughly until creamy.

3. Add the Fresh Ingredients

To the mashed avocado, add the finely chopped onion, tomatoes (if using), jalapeños or serrano peppers, and cilantro. These ingredients add crunch, spice, and a hint of freshness to the guacamole.

4. Season with Lime, Salt, and Pepper

Squeeze in the juice of 1-2 limes, adjusting based on your preference. Lime juice adds brightness and helps prevent the avocado from browning. Season generously with salt to taste and a pinch of black pepper if desired.

5. Mix and Taste

Stir all the ingredients together until well combined. Taste the guacamole and adjust the seasoning as needed, adding more lime juice, salt, or pepper to taste.

6. Serve and Garnish

Transfer the guacamole to a serving bowl and garnish with additional chopped cilantro or a sprinkle of smoked paprika or chili powder for a burst of color. Serve immediately with tortilla chips, fresh veggies, or as a topping for your favorite Mexican dishes.

Tips for Perfect Guacamole

Use Fresh Ingredients: Fresh lime juice, cilantro, and onion make all the difference in flavor, so skip the bottled lime juice and dried herbs.

Choose Ripe Avocados: Ripe avocados are key to creamy guacamole. They should yield slightly when pressed but not feel mushy or too soft.

Adjust Spice Level: For mild guacamole, remove the seeds from the jalapeños or skip them altogether. For a spicier kick, leave in some seeds or add an extra pepper.

Serve Immediately: Guacamole is best enjoyed fresh, as avocados tend to brown when exposed to air. If you need to store it, cover it with plastic wrap pressed directly onto the surface to minimize browning.

Variations of Guacamole

While traditional guacamole is simple, there are many ways to customize it to your taste:

Fruit-Infused Guacamole: Add diced mango, pineapple, or pomegranate seeds for a touch of sweetness that pairs beautifully with the creaminess of the avocado.

Roasted Garlic Guacamole: Mix in a few cloves of roasted garlic for a deep, mellow garlic flavor.

Bacon Guacamole: Top with crispy crumbled bacon for a savory twist that adds crunch.

Guacamole with Corn and Black Beans: Mix in some roasted corn kernels and black beans for extra texture and protein, creating a hearty guacamole.

Serving Suggestions

Guacamole is versatile and pairs well with many dishes:

As a Dip: Serve with tortilla chips, pita chips, or fresh veggies like carrots, bell peppers, and cucumber slices.

On Tacos and Burritos: Use guacamole as a creamy topping for tacos, burritos, or fajitas.

In Salads and Bowls: Add a scoop of guacamole to salads or grain bowls for extra flavor and healthy fats.

With Grilled Meats and Fish: Guacamole complements grilled chicken, steak, or fish, adding freshness to the meal.

The History of Guacamole

Guacamole has roots in Aztec cuisine, with the word itself derived from the Nahuatl word "āhuacamolli," which means "avocado sauce." The Aztecs prized avocados for their rich, creamy texture and nutritional value, and they combined them with simple ingredients like tomatoes and spices to create what we now know as guacamole. Today, guacamole is a staple in Mexican cuisine and has gained global popularity for its delicious flavor and health benefits.

Frequently Asked Questions

Q: How can I keep guacamole from turning brown?

To prevent browning, press plastic wrap directly onto the surface of the guacamole to minimize air exposure. Alternatively, store it in an airtight container with a layer of lime juice on top.

Q: Can I make guacamole ahead of time?

Guacamole is best enjoyed fresh, but you can make it up to a few hours in advance if needed. Store it in the refrigerator with plastic wrap pressed onto the surface.

Q: Can I use lemon juice instead of lime?

Yes, lemon juice can be used as an alternative to lime juice, though lime juice is traditionally used in Mexican guacamole for its flavor.

Q: What should I do if my avocados aren't ripe?

Place unripe avocados in a paper bag with an apple or banana to speed up ripening. The ethylene gas released by these fruits help soften the avocados.

Why You'll Love This Guacamole Recipe

This classic guacamole recipe is fresh, creamy, and bursting with flavor, capturing the authentic taste of Mexican guacamole with just a handful of ingredients. The combination of creamy avocado, tangy lime juice, and fresh cilantro makes each bite refreshing and satisfying. Whether you're serving it as a dip, adding it to your favorite Mexican dishes, or enjoying it as a snack, this guacamole recipe is sure to be a crowd-pleaser. It's quick, easy, and versatile, making it a perfect addition to any meal. Enjoy the rich, delicious flavor of homemade guacamole with this simple and authentic recipe!

27

Tamales Recipe

Tamales are a beloved Mexican dish, made with soft masa (corn dough) that's filled with a savory or sweet filling, wrapped in corn husks or banana leaves, and steamed to perfection. They're often enjoyed during holidays, family gatherings, or special occasions, where families come together to make large batches of these delicious treats. These traditional tamales recipes are both flavorful and versatile, allowing you to customize the filling and make a variety of tamales to suit your taste.

Ingredients

For the Masa:

4 cups masa harina (corn flour for tamales)

1 cup lard or vegetable shortening (traditional, but optional for a vegan version)

1 tbsp baking powder

1 tsp of salt

3 to 4 cups of warm chicken or vegetable broth (add as needed for consistency)

For the Filling (Pork, Chicken, or Vegetarian):

2 lbs. pork shoulder, chicken thighs, or a mix of vegetables (such as mushrooms and peppers)

4 dried guajillo chiles, stemmed and seeded

2 dried ancho chiles, stemmed and seeded

1 onion, chopped

3 garlic cloves, peeled

2 cups of chicken or vegetable broth

Salt and pepper to taste

For Wrapping:

30-40 dried corn husks, soaked in warm water for 1 hour to soften

Step-by-Step Instructions

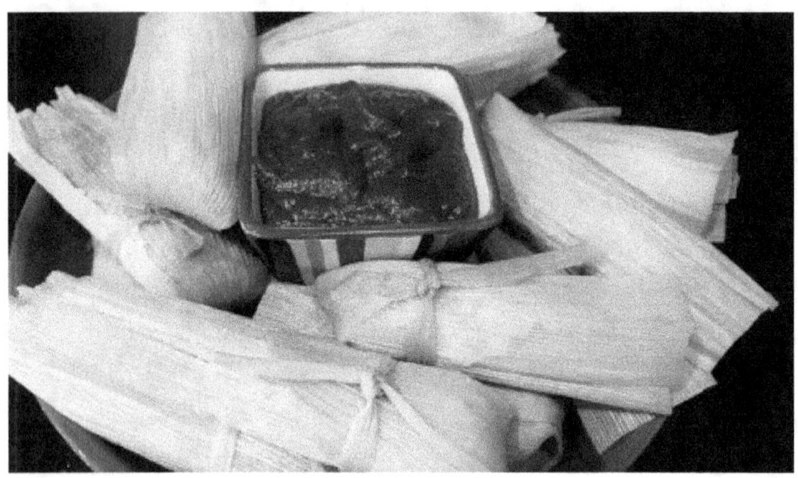

1. PREPARE THE CORN Husks

Soak the corn husks in a large bowl of warm water for at least an hour to make them pliable and easy to work with. This will help them wrap around the tamales without cracking or breaking.

2. Make the Filling

If using meat, cook the pork shoulder or chicken thighs in a pot with water until tender (about 1-2 hours for pork and 45 minutes for chicken). Shred the cooked meat with two forks.

To make the sauce, toast the dried guajillo and ancho chiles lightly in a dry skillet over medium heat, then soak them in hot water for about 15 minutes until they soften. Blend the softened chiles with the chopped onion, garlic, broth, salt, and pepper until smooth.

In a skillet, add the shredded meat or vegetables and pour in the sauce. Simmer for about 15-20 minutes, allowing the flavors to meld. Adjust seasoning as needed and set the filling aside.

3. Prepare the Masa Dough

In a large mixing bowl, beat the lard or shortening until it's light and fluffy. In a separate bowl, mix the masa harina, baking powder, and salt. Gradually add the dry mixture to the lard, alternating with warm broth, until the dough is smooth and spreadable. The masa should be soft but not too wet.

To test the dough, drop a small ball of masa into a glass of water; if it floats, it's ready. If it sinks, beat the dough a bit longer to incorporate more air.

4. Assemble the Tamales

Take a soaked corn husk and pat it dry. Spread about 2-3 tablespoons of masa dough onto the center of the husk, forming a rectangle. Add a spoonful of filling in the center of the masa.

Fold the sides of the corn husk over the filling, then fold up the bottom to enclose it, creating a small rectangular package. If needed, tie the tamale with a strip of corn husk to keep it secure.

Repeat this process with the remaining masa, filling, and corn husks.

5. Steam the Tamales

In a large steamer pot, add water just below the steamer basket. Stand the tamales upright in the steamer, with the open end facing up. Cover the tamales with a damp cloth or additional corn husks, then cover with the pot lid.

Steam over medium heat for about 1.5 to 2 hours, or until the masa pulls away easily from the corn husk. Check the water level periodically and add more hot water as needed to keep the steam going.

6. Serve and Enjoy

Once the tamales are done, let them cool slightly. Serve them in their corn husks, allowing each person to unwrap their own tamale.

Tamales are delicious on their own, or you can top them with fresh salsa, sour cream, or a squeeze of lime.

Tips for Perfect Tamales

Test the Masa: The "float test" is a great way to check if your masa is ready. If it floats, the dough is light and airy. If not, keep beating the dough.

Add Broth Gradually: Add the warm broth a little at a time to avoid a too-wet masa. The dough should be easily spreadable but hold its shape.

Pack the Tamales Snugly: Stand the tamales upright in the steamer, but don't overcrowd them. They should be packed snugly to prevent them from falling over, but with enough room for steam to circulate.

Let Them Rest: After steaming, allow the tamales to rest for a few minutes. This helps them firm up and makes them easier to unwrap.

Variations of Tamales

Tamales are incredibly versatile, and you can get creative with both the masa and filling:

Cheese and Roasted Pepper Tamales: Fill the masa with slices of cheese and roasted poblano peppers for a vegetarian option.

Sweet Tamales: Add a bit of sugar to the masa and fill with sweet ingredients like pineapple, raisins, or cinnamon for dessert tamales.

Green Chili and Chicken Tamales: Use a green tomatillo salsa for the filling with shredded chicken for a zesty alternative.

Serving Suggestions and Side Dishes

Tamales are often enjoyed with simple sides that enhance their flavors:

Mexican Rice: Fluffy Mexican rice is a perfect side that complements the flavors of tamales.

Refried Beans: Creamy refried beans add richness and are a classic pairing.

Salsa Verde or Salsa Roja: Drizzle your tamales with salsa for added flavor.

Fresh Salad: A light salad with lettuce, tomatoes, and avocado provides a refreshing contrast to the hearty tamales.

The Cultural Significance of Tamales

Tamales have been a part of Mexican cuisine for centuries, with origins dating back to the ancient civilizations of Mesoamerica, including the Aztecs and Mayans. They were traditionally prepared for celebrations, feasts, and religious ceremonies, and tamales continue to be a staple in Mexican culture, often enjoyed during holidays, family gatherings, and special occasions.

Making tamales is a labor of love that's often done as a family, with each person helping to assemble, fill, and wrap the tamales. The process itself is a time-honored tradition that brings families and communities together.

Frequently Asked Questions

Q: Can I make tamales in advance?

Yes, tamales can be made ahead of time. You can prepare the filling and masa a day in advance, then assemble and steam them the next day. You can also steam the tamales, let them cool, and reheat them in the steamer when ready to serve.

Q: Can I freeze tamales?

Yes, tamales freeze well. Place them in a freezer-safe container or bag, and freeze for up to 3 months. Reheat them in a steamer for about 20-30 minutes, or until warmed through.

Q: How do I reheat leftover tamales?

The best way to reheat tamales is by steaming them again for about 10-15 minutes. You can also microwave them wrapped in a damp paper towel, though this may slightly alter the texture.

Q: Can I use store-bought masa?

Yes, if you have access to a Mexican grocery store, fresh masa is a great shortcut. Simply mix it with a bit of lard, salt, and baking powder before using.

Why You'll Love This Tamales Recipe

These traditional tamales recipes are full of flavor, with a rich, tender masa that complements the savory filling perfectly. Making tamales is a fun and rewarding experience, allowing you to enjoy the authentic flavors of Mexican cuisine and share them with family and friends. Whether you're new to making tamales or a seasoned pro, this recipe is adaptable and can be customized with your favorite fillings. Enjoy the comfort, tradition, and delicious taste of homemade tamales with this classic recipe!

28

Churros Recipe

Churros are a classic Spanish and Mexican treat, known for their crispy exterior, soft interior, and delicious cinnamon-sugar coating. These golden-fried dough sticks are perfect for dipping in rich chocolate sauce or enjoying on their own. Churros are easy to make at home with a few simple ingredients, and they're a crowd-pleaser for any occasion—from weekend brunch to festive gatherings. This recipe guides you through creating authentic, homemade churros that are light, airy, and perfectly sweet.

Ingredients

For the Churros:

1 cup of water

2 tbsp sugar

1/2 tsp salt

2 tbsp unsalted butter

1 cup all-purpose flour

1 tsp vanilla extract

2 large eggs

Vegetable oil, for frying

For the Cinnamon-Sugar Coating:

1/2 cup of sugar

1 tsp ground cinnamon

For Chocolate Dipping Sauce (optional):

1 cup heavy cream

1 cup of semi-sweet chocolate chips

A pinch of salt

Step-by-Step Instructions

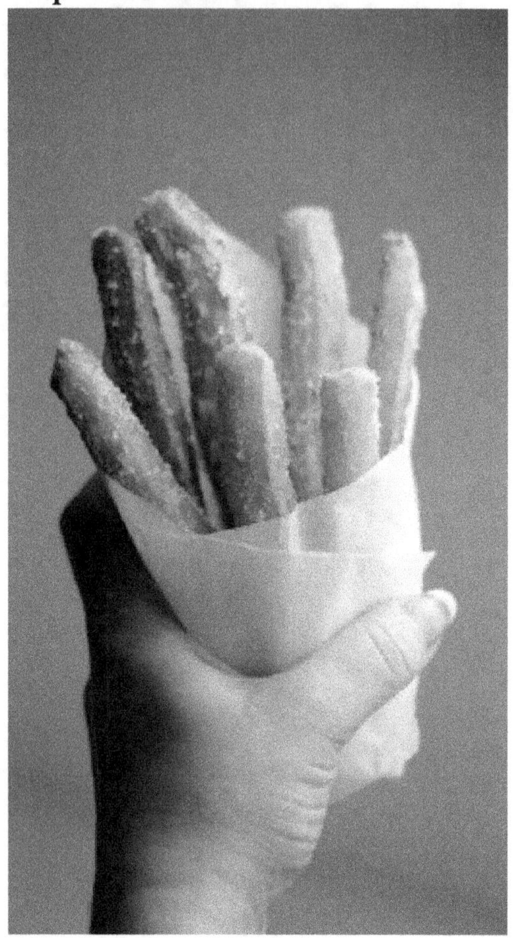

1. MAKE THE CHURRO Dough

In a medium saucepan, combine the water, sugar, salt, and butter. Bring the mixture to a boil over medium heat, stirring occasionally to melt the butter. Once the mixture reaches a boil, reduce the heat to low and add the flour all at once. Stir continuously with a wooden spoon until the dough forms a smooth ball and pulls away from the sides of the pan (about 2-3 minutes).

2. Add the Eggs and Vanilla

Remove the dough from the heat and let it cool for a few minutes. Add the vanilla extract and the eggs one at a time, mixing well after each addition. The dough will look lumpy at first but will smooth out as you continue to stir. Once the dough is smooth and well combined, transfer it to a piping bag fitted with a large star tip.

3. Heat the Oil

In a deep skillet or heavy pot, heat about 2 inches of vegetable oil to 350°F (175°C). Use a thermometer to monitor the oil temperature, as maintaining the right temperature is key to frying the churros evenly.

4. Pipe and Fry the Churros

Carefully pipe 4–6-inch strips of dough into the hot oil, cutting the end of each churro with a pair of scissors or a knife to release it from the piping bag. Fry the churros in batches, making sure not to overcrowd the pan. Fry for about 2-3 minutes per side, or until golden brown and crispy. Use a slotted spoon to transfer the churros to a paper towel-lined plate to drain excess oil.

5. Coat the Churros in Cinnamon Sugar

In a shallow dish, combine the sugar and ground cinnamon. While the churros are still warm, roll them in the cinnamon-sugar mixture until fully coated.

6. Prepare the Chocolate Dipping Sauce (Optional)

For an extra indulgent treat, prepare a rich chocolate sauce. In a small saucepan, heat the heavy cream over medium heat until it just begins to simmer. Remove from the heat, add the chocolate chips and a pinch of salt, and stir until smooth and glossy. Serve the warm churros with the chocolate sauce for dipping.

Tips for Perfect Churros

Keep the Oil Temperature Steady: Use a thermometer to keep the oil at 350°F (175°C). If the oil is too hot, the churros may brown too quickly on the outside and stay raw on the inside.

Work in Batches: Fry the churros in small batches to avoid over-crowding, which can cause uneven cooking.

Use the Right Piping Tip: A large star piping tip creates the classic churro ridges, which help the cinnamon-sugar coating stick.

Roll in Cinnamon Sugar While Warm: Coat the churros in cinnamon sugar right after frying, as the warmth helps the sugar stick.

Variations of Churros

While classic churros are delicious on their own, there are fun ways to switch things up:

Filled Churros: Once cooled, use a piping bag fitted with a small tip to fill churros with dulce de leche, chocolate, or caramel for a surprise center.

Chocolate Churros: Add 1-2 tablespoons of cocoa powder to the dough for a chocolaty twist.

Spicy Cinnamon Churros: Add a pinch of cayenne pepper to the cinnamon-sugar coating for a hint of heat that pairs wonderfully with sweetness.

Serving Suggestions

Churros are perfect for enjoying on their own or with a variety of dips:

Classic Chocolate Sauce: Dark chocolate sauce is a traditional and decadent choice.

Caramel or Dulce de Leche: A sweet, creamy caramel sauce complements the cinnamon sugar.

Fruit Dip: Try dipping churros in a fresh berry compote or a raspberry sauce for a fruity twist.

The Origin of Churros

Churros have roots in Spain and Portugal and were brought to Latin America, where they became incredibly popular. Traditional churros are often enjoyed with hot chocolate for breakfast or dessert, especially in Spain. In Mexico and other Latin American countries, churros are commonly sold by street vendors and enjoyed as a warm snack or dessert. Their simple, delicious flavor has made churros a popular treat around the world.

Frequently Asked Questions

Q: Can I make churros in advance?

Churros are best enjoyed fresh, as they tend to lose their crispiness when stored. However, you can prepare the dough ahead of time and refrigerate it for up to a day. Let the dough come to room temperature before frying.

Q: How do I reheat churros?

To reheat churros, place them in a preheated oven at 350°F (175°C) for about 5-8 minutes. Avoid microwaving, as this can make them soggy.

Q: Can I bake churros instead of frying them?

Yes, you can bake churros for a lighter option. Pipe the dough onto a parchment-lined baking sheet and bake at 400°F (200°C) for 15-20 minutes, or until golden. They may not be as crispy as fried churros, but they're still delicious.

Q: Can I freeze churros?

Yes, you can freeze unfried churro dough or freeze cooked churros. To freeze unfried dough, pipe the churros onto a tray and freeze until solid, then transfer to a freezer bag. Fry directly from frozen, adding a few extra minutes to the cooking time. To freeze cooked churros, let them cool completely, freeze, and reheat in the oven.

Why You'll Love This Churros Recipe

This churros recipe is a delightful treat that's easy to make and perfect for any occasion. The crispy exterior and soft, fluffy interior, coated with sweet cinnamon sugar, make every bite irresistible. Plus, the option to dip them in a rich chocolate sauce elevates the experience to something truly special. Whether you're making them for a celebration, sharing with family, or just enjoying a cozy treat at home, these homemade churros are sure to impress. Give this recipe a try for an authentic and delicious churro experience that brings a taste of Mexico and Spain right to your kitchen. Enjoy every warm, sweet bite!

29

Pancita Recipe

Pancita, also known as pancita de res, is a traditional Mexican soup made with beef tripe and seasoned with rich, bold spices. Often referred to as a cousin to the well-known menudo, pancita is a comforting and hearty dish that's perfect for cold days or as a weekend treat. With its rich broth, tender tripe, and savory spices, pancita is enjoyed for its depth of flavor and is often considered a restorative dish, especially for family gatherings and celebrations. This recipe provides a step-by-step guide to making authentic pancita, featuring aromatic spices and a spicy chile-based broth that brings out the best in this classic Mexican stew.

Ingredients

For the Pancita:

2 lbs. beef tripe (honeycomb tripe, well cleaned)

1 lb. beef feet (optional, for added richness)

10 cups of water

1 large onion, halved

4 garlic cloves, peeled

2 bay leaves

Salt to taste

For the Chile Broth:

4 dried guajillo chiles, stemmed and seeded

2 dried ancho chiles, stemmed and seeded

2-3 dried pasilla chiles, stemmed and seeded

1 tsp ground cumin

1 tsp dried oregano (preferably Mexican oregano)

1/2 tsp ground cloves
1/4 tsp of ground black pepper
Salt to taste
Optional Toppings:
Freshly chopped cilantro
Diced onions
Lime wedges
Crushed dried oregano
Step-by-Step Instructions

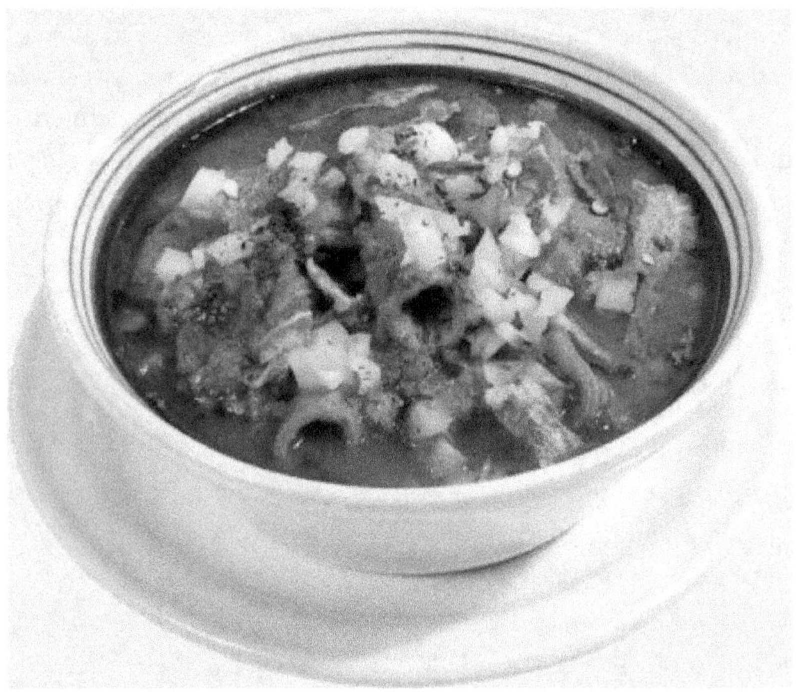

1. CLEAN AND PREPARE the Tripe

If the tripe has not been pre-cleaned, rinse it thoroughly under cold water, scrubbing gently. To help reduce the strong odor of tripe, you can briefly blanch it in a pot of boiling water for about 5 minutes, then drain and rinse it again.

Cut the tripe into small bite-sized pieces, about 1-inch squares, and set aside.

2. Cook the Tripe and Beef Feet

In a large pot, add the tripe and beef feet if using, along with 10 cups of water, the onion halves, garlic cloves, bay leaves, and a generous pinch of salt. Bring to a boil, then reduce the heat to low. Cover and simmer for about 2-3 hours, or until the tripe is tender and the broth is rich and flavorful.

As the soup simmers, skim off any foam or impurities that rise to the top.

3. Prepare the Chile Broth

While the tripe is cooking, prepare the chile broth. Toast the guajillo, ancho, and pasilla chiles in a dry skillet over medium heat for about 30 seconds on each side, until they become fragrant. Be careful not to burn them.

Transfer the toasted chiles to a bowl and cover with hot water. Let them soak for 15 minutes, or until they soften. Once softened, place the chiles in a blender along with 1 cup of soaking liquid, cumin, oregano, ground cloves, black pepper, and a pinch of salt. Blend until smooth.

4. Combine the Chile Broth and Soup

Once the tripe is tender, remove the onion, garlic, and bay leaves from the pot. Pour the chile mixture into the pot with the tripe and stir to combine. Taste the broth and adjust the seasoning as needed with salt and additional spices.

Simmer the soup for another 20-30 minutes to allow the flavors to meld together.

5. Serve the Pancita

Ladle the hot pancita into bowls, ensuring each bowl has plenty of tripe and flavorful broth. Serve with fresh toppings like chopped cilantro, diced onions, and a squeeze of lime juice. Crushed dried oregano can also be sprinkled on top for an extra layer of flavor.

Pancita is best enjoyed with warm corn tortillas on the side, perfect for dipping into the broth.

Tips for Perfect Pancita

Clean the Tripe Thoroughly: Tripe has a unique aroma, so it's essential to clean it well. Blanching helps remove any residual odor and makes it more palatable.

Adjust the Spice Level: The chiles in the broth add flavor and mild heat. If you prefer spicier pancita, add a few arbol chiles to the mix.

Cook Low and Slow: Tripe benefits from slow cooking, so give it time to become tender. A slow-cooked pancita has a rich, flavorful broth that can't be rushed.

Use Mexican Oregano: Mexican oregano has a distinct, earthy flavor that pairs well with the spices in pancita. It can be found in most Latin grocery stores.

Variations of Pancita

Pancita is versatile and can be customized in different ways:

Pancita Verde: Use a green sauce made from tomatillos, green chiles, and cilantro for a variation that's lighter and tangier than the traditional red chile version.

Add Hominy: Add hominy (large corn kernels) for added texture and flavor, like menudo.

Make it Spicier: For those who enjoy a spicy kick, add diced jalapeños or serrano peppers as a garnish, or include a few arbol chiles in the chile broth.

Serving Suggestions

Pancita is best enjoyed with simple sides and garnishes:

Warm Corn Tortillas: Soft corn tortillas are perfect for soaking up the flavorful broth.

Fresh Salsa or Hot Sauce: Add a dollop of salsa or a drizzle of hot sauce for a spicier bite.

Mexican Rice: A side of Mexican rice can be a hearty addition to the meal.

Lime and Cilantro: Fresh lime wedges and cilantro add brightness and balance the richness of the soup.

The Cultural Significance of Pancita

Pancita is a dish with deep roots in Mexican cuisine, traditionally enjoyed for its nourishing and restorative qualities. Like Menudo, it is often served during gatherings or as a weekend treat and is considered a go-to meal for celebrations and family gatherings. In some regions, pancita is also enjoyed as a hangover remedy due to its richness and the perceived revitalizing effects of the broth and spices.

Making pancita at home can be a labor of love, as it requires time and patience, but it's well worth the effort to bring this comforting, flavorful dish to the table.

Frequently Asked Questions

Q: Can I make pancita without beef feet?

Yes, you can make pancita without beef feet. The beef feet add richness to the broth, but if you prefer, you can omit them or replace them with beef bones for added flavor.

Q: How long does pancita last in the refrigerator?

Pancita can be stored in the refrigerator for up to 3-4 days in an airtight container. Reheat on the stove for the best flavor and texture.

Q: Can I freeze pancita?

Yes, pancita freezes well. Store it in freezer-safe containers for up to 3 months. Thaw in the refrigerator overnight and reheat gently on the stove.

Q: Can I make pancita in a slow cooker?

Yes, after preparing the tripe and broth, you can transfer everything to a slow cooker and cook on low for 6-8 hours, or until the tripe is tender.

Why You'll Love This Pancita Recipe

This pancita recipe is a comforting, flavorful way to experience traditional Mexican cuisine. The slow-cooked tripe, rich broth, and bold spices create a soup that's not only nourishing but also packed with depth and character. Whether you're enjoying it as a family meal, a weekend treat, or sharing it with friends, pancita is a dish that brings warmth and connection to the table. Enjoy the rich flavors, cultural history, and heartwarming experience of homemade pancita with this easy-to-follow recipe. With a few ingredients and a bit of time, you'll create a delicious, authentic Mexican stew that's sure to satisfy.

30

Tres Leches Cake Recipe

Tres leches cake is a classic Latin American dessert made by soaking a soft sponge cake in a rich, three-milk mixture. The name tres leches translates to "three milks" in Spanish, referring to the blend of condensed milk, evaporated milk, and heavy cream that gives this cake its signature moist texture and deliciously creamy flavor. Light, airy, and incredibly indulgent, tres leches cake is perfect for special occasions, gatherings, or any time you crave a sweet treat. This recipe provides a step-by-step guide to making the ultimate tres leches cake, complete with a whipped cream topping for an extra touch of decadence.

Ingredients

For the Cake:

1 cup all-purpose flour

1 1/2 tsp baking powder

1/4 tsp salt

5 large eggs, separated

1 cup sugar, divided

1/3 cup whole milk

1 tsp vanilla extract

For the Three-Milk Mixture:

1 can (14 oz) sweetened condensed milk

1 can (12 oz) evaporated milk

1/4 cup heavy cream

For the Whipped Cream Topping:

1 cup heavy whipping cream

3 tbsp powdered sugar

1/2 tsp vanilla extract

Optional Toppings:

Fresh berries or sliced strawberries

A sprinkle of cinnamon

Toasted coconut flakes

Step-by-Step Instructions

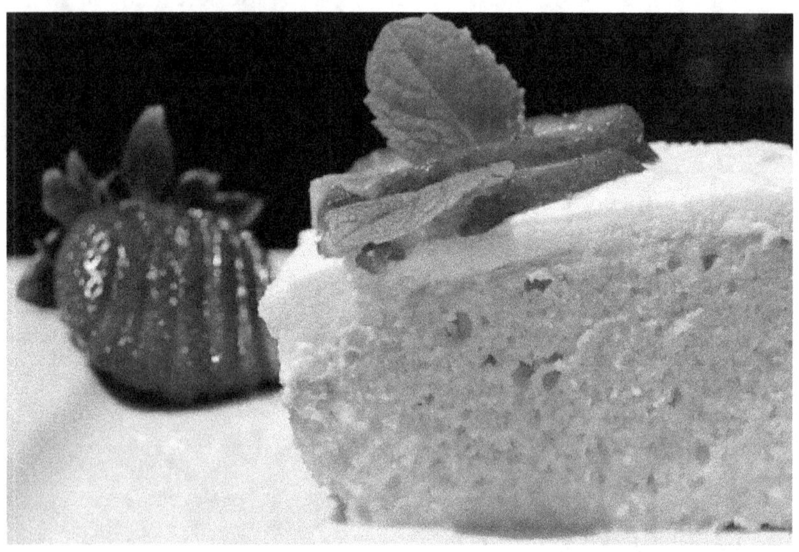

1. PREHEAT THE OVEN and Prepare the Baking Dish

Preheat your oven to 350°F (175°C). Grease and flour a 9x13-inch baking dish to prevent the cake from sticking.

2. Make the Cake Batter

In a medium bowl, whisk together the flour, baking powder, and salt. Set aside.

In a large bowl, beat the egg yolks with 3/4 cup of sugar until the mixture is light and fluffy. Add the milk and vanilla extract, mix until combined.

In a separate bowl, beat the egg whites on high speed until soft peaks form. Gradually add the remaining 1/4 cup of sugar and continue to beat until stiff peaks form. Gently fold the egg whites into the egg yolk mixture. Add the dry ingredients to the egg mixture, folding gently until just combined. Be careful not to overmix, as you want the batter to stay light and airy.

3. Bake the Cake

Pour the batter into the prepared baking dish and spread it evenly. Bake for 25-30 minutes, or until a toothpick inserted into the center of the cake comes out clean. The cake should be golden on top.

Allow the cake to cool completely in the pan.

4. Prepare the Three-Milk Mixture

In a mixing bowl, whisk together the sweetened condensed milk, evaporated milk, and heavy cream until well combined.

5. Soak the Cake

Once the cake has cooled, use a fork or a skewer to poke holes all over the surface. Slowly pour the three-milk mixture over the cake, making sure it soaks evenly. The holes will help the cake absorb the milk mixture, making it extra moist.

Cover the cake and refrigerate for at least 1 hour, or preferably overnight. The longer it sits, the more flavorful and moister the cake will become.

6. Make the Whipped Cream Topping

Just before serving, prepare the whipped cream topping. In a large bowl, beat the heavy whipping cream, powdered sugar, and vanilla extract on high speed until soft peaks form.

Spread the whipped cream evenly over the top of the cake.

7. Garnish and Serve

Add your choice of toppings, such as fresh berries, a sprinkle of cinnamon, or toasted coconut flakes, for extra flavor and presentation. Slice and serve the cake cold, straight from the fridge.

Tips for Perfect Tres Leches Cake

Use Room Temperature Eggs: Room temperature eggs create a better texture in the cake and make it easier to whip the egg whites.

Fold Gently: When mixing the egg whites into the batter, use a gentle folding motion to keep the batter light and airy.

Let It Soak: For the best flavor, let the cake soak in the milk mixture for at least 4 hours, or ideally overnight. This allows the cake to absorb all the liquid and develop a rich, creamy texture.

Serve Cold: Tres leches cake is best served chilled, as the cool temperature enhances the cake's creamy texture.

Variations of Tres Leches Cake

While the classic tres leches cake is delicious as is, you can get creative with different flavors and additions:

Coconut Tres Leches Cake: Substitute some of the heavy cream with coconut milk for a tropical twist. Garnish with toasted coconut flakes for extra flavor.

Chocolate Tres Leches Cake: Add 1/4 cup of cocoa powder to the dry ingredients for a chocolaty version of the classic dessert.

Coffee Tres Leches Cake: Add a tablespoon of instant coffee to the milk mixture for a coffee-flavored variation that pairs well with chocolate or caramel.

Serving Suggestions and Toppings

Tres leches cake is often enjoyed with various toppings that add flavor and texture:

Fresh Berries: Strawberries, raspberries, and blueberries add a fresh contrast to the creamy cake.

Cinnamon: A light dusting of cinnamon enhances the flavor of the cake and adds a touch of warmth.

Caramel Drizzle: Drizzle caramel sauce over the whipped cream topping for an extra layer of indulgence.

Toasted Nuts: Chopped toasted almonds, pecans, or walnuts add a bit of crunch.

The History of Tres Leches Cake

Tres leches cake has a rich history in Latin American cuisine, with origins that trace back to countries like Mexico, Nicaragua, and

Costa Rica. Some believe it was inspired by European milk-soaked cakes like trifle, but tres leches cake gained popularity in Latin America, where it became a beloved dessert at celebrations and gatherings. The simple ingredients and deliciously moist texture of tres leches cake have made it a staple dessert throughout Latin America and beyond.

Frequently Asked Questions

Q: How long can tres leches cake be stored?

Tres leches cake can be stored in the refrigerator, covered, for up to 4-5 days. The cake may continue to absorb the milk mixture, making it even moister over time.

Q: Can I make tres leches cake in advance?

Yes, tres leches cake is best made a day ahead, as this gives the cake plenty of time to soak up the milk mixture. Prepare the whipped cream topping just before serving for the freshest taste.

Q: Can I freeze tres leches cake?

It's not recommended to freeze tres leches cake because the texture can become mushy after thawing. However, you can freeze the plain cake (before soaking it in milk) and add the milk mixture once it's thawed.

Q: Can I make this recipe gluten-free?

Yes, you can use a gluten-free all-purpose flour blend in place of regular flour. Ensure all other ingredients are gluten-free as well.

Why You'll Love This Tres Leches Cake Recipe

This tres leches cake recipe is the perfect balance of sweet, creamy, and light flavors that melt in your mouth. The soft sponge cake soaks up the three-milk mixture beautifully, resulting in a texture that's moist without being overly heavy. Topped with fresh whipped cream and your choice of garnish, each bite is a delightful combination of creamy richness and light sweetness. Tres leches cake is ideal for celebrations, holidays, or any time you're in the mood for a special treat. Its simple ingredients and impressive taste make it a crowd-pleaser that's sure to become a favorite. Enjoy this classic Latin American dessert that brings comfort, sweetness, and a touch of elegance to any occasion!

31

Chilaquiles Recipe

Chilaquiles is a traditional Mexican dish made with fried tortilla chips simmered in a delicious, flavorful sauce and topped with fresh ingredients like cheese, crema, onions, and sometimes eggs or shredded chicken. It's often enjoyed as a hearty breakfast or brunch dish and is perfect for using up leftover tortillas. With its saucy, crispy, and cheesy elements, chilaquiles is comforting, filling, and bursting with authentic Mexican flavors. This recipe will guide you through making classic chilaquiles with either red or green sauce, giving you options to customize the dish to your liking.

Ingredients

For the Chilaquiles:

12 corn tortillas, cut into quarters

Vegetable oil, for frying

Salt, to taste

For the Red or Green Sauce:

Red Sauce:

4 dried guajillo chiles, stemmed and seeded

2 dried ancho chiles, stemmed and seeded

1 large tomato, chopped

1/2 onion, chopped

2 garlic cloves

Salt, to taste

Green Sauce:

10-12 tomatillos, husked and rinsed

1/2 onion, chopped

1-2 jalapeños or serrano peppers, seeded for less heat

2 garlic cloves

Fresh cilantro, a small handful

Salt, to taste

Optional Toppings:

1/2 cup crumbled queso fresco or shredded cheese

Mexican crema or sour cream

Sliced avocado

Fried or scrambled eggs

Shredded chicken (optional)

Fresh cilantro, chopped

Thinly sliced red onion

Step-by-Step Instructions

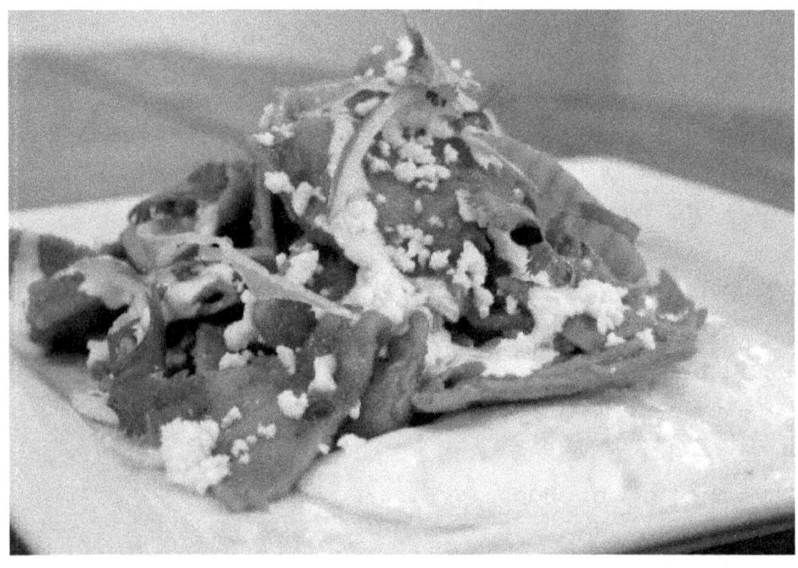

1. PREPARE THE TORTILLA Chips

In a large skillet, heat about 1/4 inch of vegetable oil over medium heat. Once hot, fry the tortilla quarters in batches until crispy and golden brown on both sides. Use a slotted spoon to transfer the chips to a paper towel-lined plate and sprinkle with a little salt while they're still warm. Set aside.

Alternatively, you can bake the tortilla chips for a lighter option. Spread them in a single layer on a baking sheet, brush lightly with oil, and bake at 350°F (175°C) for about 10-15 minutes, or until crispy.

2. Make the Red or Green Sauce

For Red Sauce: Toast the guajillo and ancho chiles lightly in a dry skillet over medium heat, being careful not to burn them. Then, place them in a bowl of hot water and let them soak for about 15 minutes until softened. In a blender, add the soaked chiles, chopped tomato, onion, garlic, and a pinch of salt. Blend until smooth, adding a little of the soaking liquid if necessary.

For Green Sauce: Place the tomatillos, onion, peppers, and garlic in a pot and cover with water. Bring to a boil and simmer for about 10 minutes, until the tomatillos are softened. Drain the water and add the cooked ingredients to a blender along with fresh cilantro and salt. Blend until smooth.

Once blended, pour the sauce into a skillet and simmer for 10-15 minutes, stirring occasionally, until the sauce thickens slightly.

3. Combine the Chips and Sauce

In the skillet with the sauce, add the fried tortilla chips and gently toss to coat them in the sauce. Let the chips simmer in the sauce for just a minute or two, until they begin to soften but still have some texture. The ideal chilaquiles have a mix of slightly crispy and soft chips, so avoid letting them soak too long.

4. Serve and Garnish

Transfer the chilaquiles to plates and top with your choice of garnishes, such as crumbled queso fresco, a drizzle of crema, sliced avocado, and fresh cilantro. For a heartier meal, add a fried egg or shredded chicken on top.

Serve immediately, as chilaquiles are best enjoyed fresh while the chips still have some crispiness.

Tips for Perfect Chilaquiles

Don't Overcook the Chips in Sauce: To maintain the best texture, coat the chips in the sauce just before serving so they don't become too soft.

Adjust the Heat Level: Use more or fewer jalapeños, serranos, or dried chiles depending on your heat preference. Removing the seeds will also reduce spiciness.

Serve Fresh: Chilaquiles are best enjoyed fresh, as the chips tend to lose their crispiness if left too long in the sauce.

Customize the Toppings: Chilaquiles can be topped with a variety of ingredients, so feel free to add what you like best, from fried eggs and avocado to spicy salsa and fresh herbs.

Variations of Chilaquiles

Chilaquiles can be customized to suit your taste preferences, making them incredibly versatile:

Chilaquiles Verdes: Use the green tomatillo sauce for a tangy and bright variation.

Chilaquiles Rojos: Use the red chile sauce for a smoky and slightly spicy flavor.

Chilaquiles con Pollo: Add shredded, cooked chicken to the chilaquiles for a more filling dish.

Chilaquiles with Eggs: Top with fried or scrambled eggs for a hearty breakfast option.

Serving Suggestions

Chilaquiles are a complete meal on their own, but you can also serve them with other sides for a more robust brunch or breakfast:

Refried Beans: Serve a side of creamy refried beans to complement the saucy chilaquiles.

Mexican Rice: A small side of Mexican rice adds flavor and makes the meal more filling.

Fresh Salsa: A fresh salsa, like pico de gallo, can add a refreshing contrast.

Sliced Avocado or Guacamole: Creamy avocado balances the spicy flavors in chilaquiles.

The Origins of Chilaquiles

Chilaquiles have their origins in traditional Mexican cuisine, where leftover tortillas were commonly repurposed into new meals. The name "chilaquiles" is derived from the Nahuatl word "chīlāquil-itl," which means "herbs or greens in chili broth." Chilaquiles were created as a way to use up day-old tortillas, turning them into a flavorful and filling dish with the addition of sauces and toppings. Today, chilaquiles are enjoyed across Mexico and are especially popular for breakfast or brunch.

Frequently Asked Questions

Q: Can I make chilaquiles ahead of time?

Chilaquiles are best enjoyed fresh, but you can make the sauce in advance and store it in the refrigerator for up to 3 days. When ready to serve, reheat the sauce and toss with freshly fried or baked tortilla chips.

Q: Can I use store-bought tortilla chips?

Yes, you can use store-bought tortilla chips for convenience. Just make sure to choose thick, sturdy chips, as they hold up better in the sauce.

Q: Are chilaquiles spicy?

The spice level of chilaquiles depends on the sauce. If you prefer a milder version, reduce or omit the hot peppers or chiles in the sauce.

Q: What's the difference between chilaquiles and nachos?

While both dishes use tortilla chips as a base, nachos are typically topped with cheese, salsa, and various toppings and baked, while chilaquiles involve simmering the chips in a sauce until they soften slightly.

Why You'll Love This Chilaquiles Recipe

This chilaquiles recipe captures the authentic flavors of Mexico, with a perfectly balanced sauce and crispy tortilla chips that soften slightly for a deliciously satisfying texture. The combination of red or green sauce with fresh toppings like cheese, crema, and avocado makes every bite full of flavor and texture.

Whether you're making them for a weekend brunch, a special breakfast, or simply to enjoy a taste of traditional Mexican cuisine, chilaquiles are a dish that brings comfort and satisfaction with every bite. Enjoy these saucy, crispy, and irresistible chilaquiles, and savor the rich flavors and traditions of this classic Mexican recipe!

32

Pozole Recipe

Pozole is a traditional Mexican soup that's rich, comforting, and full of vibrant flavors. Made with tender pork (or sometimes chicken), hominy, and a deeply flavorful broth, pozole is enjoyed during holidays, family gatherings, and special occasions. There are three main types of pozole: pozole rojo (red pozole), pozole verde (green pozole), and pozole blanco (white pozole), each with its unique flavor profile and color. This recipe will guide you through making classic pozole rojo, with a smoky, spicy red chile broth that's balanced by fresh, colorful garnishes. Pozole is a meal, with layers of flavor and texture that make it an unforgettable dish.

Ingredients

For the Pozole:

2 lbs. pork shoulder, cut into large chunks (or substitute chicken if preferred)

1 lb. pork bones (optional, for added flavor)

10 cups water or low-sodium chicken broth

1 large onion, halved

5 garlic cloves

1 bay leaf

Salt, to taste

1 can (25 oz) hominy, drained and rinsed

For the Red Chile Sauce:

4 dried guajillo chiles, stemmed and seeded

2 dried ancho chiles, stemmed and seeded

2-3 dried pasilla chiles, stemmed and seeded

1/2 tsp ground cumin

1/2 tsp dried oregano (preferably Mexican oregano)

Salt, to taste

Optional Toppings:

Shredded cabbage or lettuce

Thinly sliced radishes

Diced white onion

Freshly chopped cilantro

Lime wedges

Avocado slices

Crushed tortilla chips or tostadas

Step-by-Step Instructions

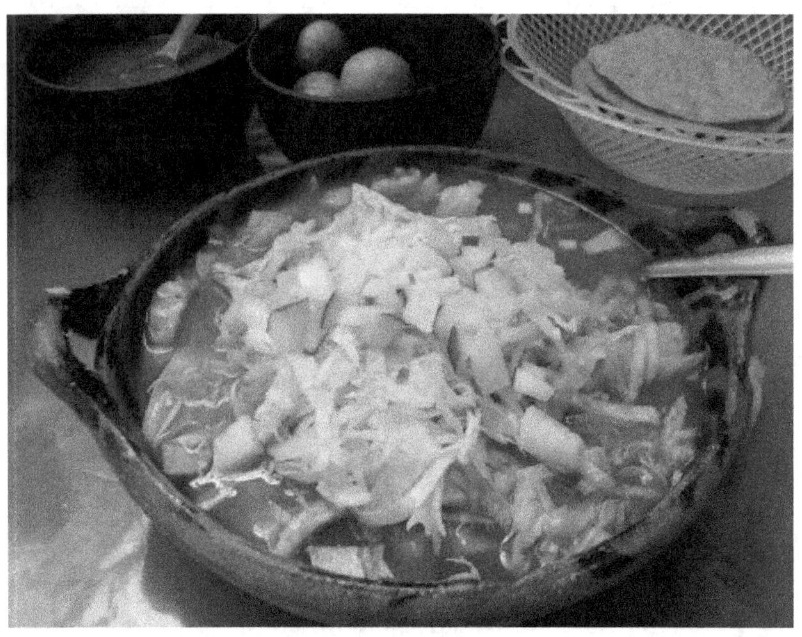

1. PREPARE THE PORK Broth

In a large pot, add the pork shoulder, pork bones (if using), water or broth, onion halves, garlic cloves, bay leaf, and a pinch of salt. Bring the mixture to a boil, then reduce the heat to low and let it simmer for about 1.5 to 2 hours, or until the pork is tender and easy to shred.

As the broth cooks, skim off any foam or impurities that rise to the surface to keep the broth clear.

2. Prepare the Red Chile Sauce

While the pork is cooking, prepare the red chile sauce. Toast the guajillo, ancho, and pasilla chiles in a dry skillet over medium heat for about 30 seconds on each side, until they become fragrant. Be careful not to burn them, as this can make the sauce bitter.

Transfer the toasted chiles to a bowl and cover them with hot water. Let them soak for about 15 minutes, or until they soften. Once softened, place the chiles in a blender along with a little soaking liquid, cumin, oregano, and a pinch of salt. Blend until smooth, adding more of the soaking liquid if needed to achieve sauce-like consistency.

3. Combine the Chile Sauce and Broth

Once the pork is tender, remove it from the pot and shred it into bite-sized pieces. Discard the onion, garlic, and bay leaf from the broth.

Strain the red chile sauce to remove any leftover seeds or skin, then pour it into the pot with the broth. Add the shredded pork back into the pot, along with the hominy, and stir to combine. Taste the broth and adjust seasoning as needed with more salt or spices.

4. Simmer the Pozole

Let the pozole simmer for another 30 minutes to allow the flavors to meld. The hominy will soften slightly, and the broth will become rich and flavorful.

5. Serve and Garnish

Ladle the hot pozole into bowls and top with your favorite garnishes. Popular toppings include shredded cabbage or lettuce, thinly sliced radishes, diced onion, chopped cilantro, and a squeeze of lime juice. Serve with crispy tostadas or crushed tortilla chips for added crunch.

Enjoy your pozole warm and with plenty of toppings!

Tips for Perfect Pozole

Choose Quality Pork: Pork shoulder is ideal for pozole as it becomes tender with long cooking, adding richness to the broth.

Adjust the Spice Level: Pozole rojo is mildly spicy, but if you prefer more heat, add a few arbol chiles to the red chile sauce.

Let It Simmer: The longer pozole simmers, the more the flavors develop. If you have time, let it cook for another hour after adding the chile sauce.

Customize with Toppings: The toppings are essential in pozole, adding fresh, crunchy, and tangy elements that balance the rich, spicy broth.

Variations of Pozole

While pozole rojo is popular, there are other types of pozole to explore:

Pozole Verde: This version uses green ingredients like tomatillos, green chiles, and fresh herbs, creating a tangy and fresh flavor profile. It's popular in regions like Guerrero, Mexico.

Pozole Blanco: This is a simpler version with a clear broth, without the addition of chiles. The flavors come from meat and hominy, and it's often served with a variety of toppings.

Chicken Pozole: Substitute the pork with chicken thighs for a lighter version of pozole. It's equally delicious and requires a shorter cooking time.

Serving Suggestions

Pozole is a complete meal on its own but pairs well with traditional sides and drinks:

Tostadas: Serve with tostadas on the side or broken into the soup for added crunch.

Mexican Rice: A side of Mexican rice complements the flavors of pozole.

Agua Fresca: Refreshing drinks like horchata or tamarind agua fresca make a great accompaniment.

Salsa and Chips: Offer extra salsa or hot sauce for those who want more spice.

The Cultural Significance of Pozole

Pozole has deep roots in Mexican culture, dating back to pre-Hispanic times when it was prepared for special ceremonies and celebrations. In ancient Mesoamerica, it was believed to be a sacred dish, enjoyed by the Aztecs and prepared with unique ritualistic significance. Today, pozole is still a beloved dish, often served during holidays like Mexican Independence Day, Christmas, and New Year's Eve, bringing families together for a hearty and comforting meal.

Making pozole at home is a time-honored tradition that families enjoy together, with each person helping to prepare, cook, and garnish the dish. It's a symbol of Mexican heritage, culture, and the joy of sharing a meal with loved ones.

Frequently Asked Questions

Q: Can I make pozole ahead of time?

Yes, pozole can be made a day in advance, which improves the flavor as it sits. Store it in the refrigerator and reheat it on the stove, adding a little broth or water if needed.

Q: How long does pozole last in the refrigerator?

Pozole will keep in the refrigerator for up to 4 days in an airtight container. Reheat gently on the stove.

Q: Can I freeze pozole?

Yes, pozole freezes well. Freeze it in freezer-safe containers for up to 3 months. Thaw in the refrigerator overnight before reheating.

Q: Where can I find hominy?

Hominy can be found in the canned goods section of most grocery stores, especially in Latin or international aisles. You can also find dried hominy, but it will need to be soaked and cooked before adding to the soup.

Why You'll Love This Pozole Recipe

This pozole recipe is a warm, flavorful, and satisfying dish that's perfect for any occasion. With tender pork, hearty hominy, and a deeply seasoned broth, each bowl is packed with authentic Mexican flavors. The toppings bring freshness, color, and texture to the dish, making every bite an exciting experience. Whether you're new to pozole or revisiting a beloved family tradition, this recipe is a true taste of Mexican comfort food. Enjoy the richness of the broth, the tenderness of the pork, and the joy of garnishing your bowl with fresh, flavorful toppings. This pozole recipe is sure to become a favorite that you'll want to make again and again.

33

Tacos al Pastor Recipe

Tacos al pastor are a beloved Mexican street food with a unique blend of smoky, spicy, and tangy flavors. Originating from Lebanese immigrants who brought shawarma-style cooking to Mexico, al pastor is made with thin slices of marinated pork that are traditionally cooked on a vertical spit, much like Middle Eastern shawarma or Greek gyro. The pork is marinated in a combination of spices, achiote paste, and pineapple, then layered with a mix of charred edges and tender, juicy meat. This homemade version gives you all the flavors of classic tacos al pastor without the need for a spit.

Ingredients

For the Marinade:

2 lbs. pork shoulder, thinly sliced

4 dried guajillo chiles, stemmed and seeded

1/4 cup achiote paste

1/4 cup fresh pineapple juice

1/4 cup of orange juice

1/4 cup of apple cider vinegar

3 garlic cloves

1/2 onion, chopped

1 tsp dried oregano (preferably Mexican oregano)

1/2 tsp ground cumin

1/2 tsp ground black pepper

1/4 tsp ground cloves (optional)

Salt to taste

For Cooking:

1/2 cup fresh pineapple, cut into small pieces

Vegetable oil, for cooking

For Serving:

Corn tortillas, warmed

Fresh cilantro, chopped

Diced white onion

Lime wedges

Optional Toppings:

Sliced avocado

Fresh salsa

Crumbled queso fresco

Step-by-Step Instructions

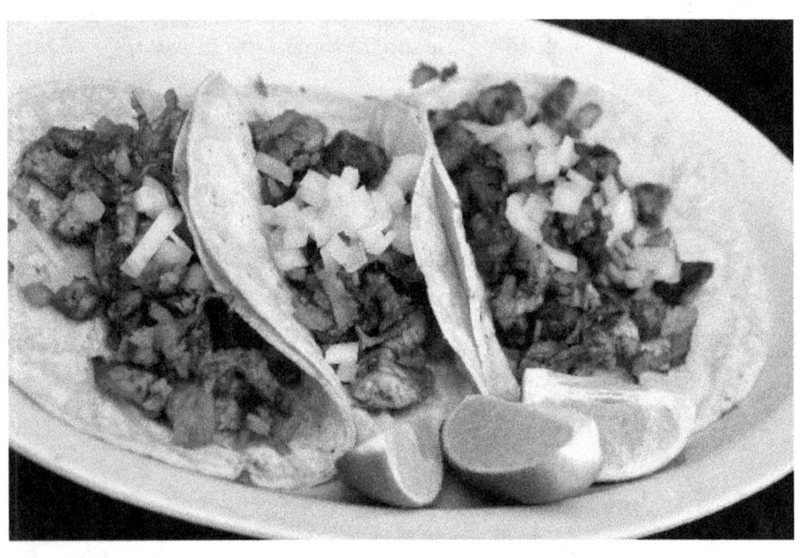

1. PREPARE THE MARINADE

Start by softening the guajillo chiles. Place them in a bowl and cover with hot water, allowing them to soak for about 15 minutes, or until they're soft. Drain and transfer them to a blender.

In the blender, add the achiote paste, pineapple juice, orange juice, apple cider vinegar, garlic, onion, oregano, cumin, black pepper, ground cloves (if using), and a pinch of salt. Blend until you have a smooth marinade.

2. Marinate the Pork

Place the thinly sliced pork shoulder in a large bowl or zip-top bag. Pour the marinade over the pork, making sure each slice is thoroughly coated. Cover and refrigerate for at least 4 hours, or ideally overnight, to allow the flavors to fully penetrate the meat.

3. Cook the Pork

If you don't have a vertical spit, you can cook the pork in a skillet. Heat a little vegetable oil in a large skillet or cast-iron pan over medium-high heat. Add the marinated pork slices in a single layer, cooking them in batches to avoid overcrowding. Sear each piece until it's caramelized and slightly charred, about 3-4 minutes per side.

Once all the pork is cooked, add the small pineapple pieces to the skillet and cook until they're caramelized and slightly charred, for about 2 minutes. This gives the pineapple a smoky, sweet flavor that pairs perfectly with the pork.

4. Chop the Pork

Once the pork is cooked and slightly cooled, chop it into small, bite-sized pieces. This gives the tacos their traditional texture with a mix of tender and crispy pork bits.

5. Warm the Tortillas

Warm the corn tortillas on a skillet or griddle until they're soft and pliable. This step is crucial for authentic tacos al pastor, as it makes the tortillas more flavorful and easier to handle.

6. Assemble the Tacos

Place a generous spoonful of chopped pork on each warm tortilla. Top with a few pieces of caramelized pineapple, a sprinkle of chopped cilantro, diced onion, and a squeeze of fresh lime juice. Serve with additional lime wedges and any optional toppings you like.

Tips for Perfect Tacos al Pastor

Slice the Pork Thinly: Thin slices cook more evenly and give the meat a tender texture with plenty of caramelized edges.

Marinate Overnight: For the most flavor, let the pork marinate for at least 8 hours or overnight.

Use Fresh Pineapple: The pineapple adds a sweet and tangy flavor that complements the savory pork. Cooking it slightly before adding it to the tacos enhances its natural sweetness.

Char the Meat: Charring the pork and pineapple adds a smoky flavor that's characteristic of traditional al pastor.

Variations of Tacos al Pastor

While the classic al pastor recipe is delicious on its own, there are several ways to adapt the recipe to your taste:

Chicken al Pastor: Substitute pork with thinly sliced chicken thighs or breasts for a lighter option.

Vegetarian al Pastor: Use portobello mushrooms or jackfruit as a meat substitute. Marinate them in the same al pastor marinade for a similar smoky, spicy flavor.

Spicy al Pastor: For extra heat, add a few chipotle peppers to the marinade or serve the tacos with a spicy salsa.

Serving Suggestions

Tacos al pastor are best served with fresh and flavorful sides:

Mexican Street Corn (Elote): Grilled corn on the cob topped with mayo, cheese, and chili powder makes a delicious side.

Mexican Rice: A simple, flavorful Mexican rice pairs wonderfully with the tacos.

Guacamole: A bowl of fresh guacamole adds creaminess and balances the spice in the tacos.

Refried Beans: Serve refried beans on the side or spread a little inside the tortilla for added flavor.

The Origins of Tacos al Pastor

Tacos al pastor have a fascinating history rooted in Mexico's multicultural influence. Lebanese immigrants who came to Mexico in the early 20th century brought with them the tradition of spit-roasting meat, which led to the creation of a uniquely Mexican take on shawarma. Instead of lamb, Mexican cooks used pork and marinated it in traditional Mexican flavors, including achiote and pineapple. The result was tacos al pastor, now a staple in Mexican street food culture and beloved worldwide.

Frequently Asked Questions

Q: Can I use store-bought achiote paste?

Yes, store-bought achiote paste is convenient and works well for this recipe. It adds the earthy, slightly sweet flavor and red color that are characteristic of al pastor.

Q: Can I grill the pork instead of pan-frying?

Yes, grilling is a great option! Marinate the pork as directed, then cook the thin slices on a hot grill until they're caramelized and slightly charred.

Q: What type of tortillas should I use?

Corn tortillas are traditional for tacos al pastor, as they add an authentic flavor and texture. If you prefer, you can also use small flour tortillas.

Q: Can I make tacos al pastor in advance?

You can marinate the pork a day in advance and cook it just before serving. However, tacos al pastor are best enjoyed fresh for the perfect balance of tender meat and crisp edges.

Why You'll Love This Tacos al Pastor Recipe

These tacos al pastor recipe brings all the smoky, spicy, and sweet flavors of a classic Mexican street food experience right to your kitchen. With its rich marinade, tender pork, and caramelized pineapple, each bite is a balance of savory, spicy, and tangy flavors. The fresh toppings add crunch and freshness, while the warm corn tortillas bring everything together. Perfect for taco night, parties, or anytime you're craving something truly special, these tacos al pastor are easy to make at home and offer an authentic taste of Mexico. En-

joy the flavors, the vibrant colors, and the satisfying texture of homemade tacos al pastor!

34

Tostadas Recipe

Tostadas are a delicious Mexican dish featuring a crisp corn tortilla base topped with a variety of flavorful ingredients. Think of them as an open-faced taco with endless topping possibilities—from refried beans and shredded chicken to guacamole and fresh veggies. Tostadas are versatile, easy to prepare, and perfect for any meal. This recipe will guide you through making the classic tostada base and give your ideas for delicious toppings, so you can customize your tostadas just the way you like.

Ingredients

For the Tostada Base:

8 small corn tortillas

Vegetable oil, for frying (or you can bake them for a lighter option)

Salt, to taste

Suggested Toppings:

Refried beans (homemade or canned)

Shredded lettuce or cabbage

Shredded chicken, ground beef, or shredded beef

Guacamole or sliced avocado

Diced tomatoes

Diced onions

Fresh cilantro, chopped

Crumbled queso fresco or shredded cheese

Mexican crema or sour cream

Hot sauce or salsa

Lime wedges for garnish
Step-by-Step Instructions

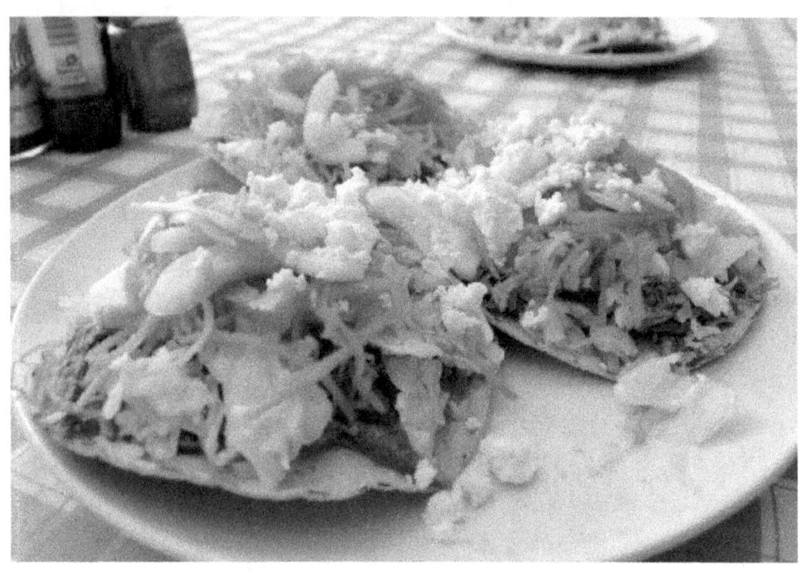

1. PREPARE THE TOSTADA Base

To make the tostada base, you can either fry or bake the corn tortillas until they're crispy.

Frying:

In a large skillet, heat about 1/4 inch of vegetable oil over medium-high heat. Once the oil is hot, carefully add one tortilla at a time, frying for about 1-2 minutes on each side, or until golden and crispy. Use tongs to transfer the tortilla to a paper towel-lined plate to drain any excess oil, and sprinkle with a little salt. Repeat with the remaining tortillas.

Baking:

Preheat your oven to 400°F (200°C). Brush each tortilla lightly with oil and place them on a baking sheet in a single layer. Bake for about 8-10 minutes, flipping halfway through, until the tortillas are crisp and golden. Sprinkle with salt while they're still warm.

2. Prepare Your Toppings

While the tostadas are cooling, prepare your desired toppings. Here are some classic options:

Refried Beans: Warm up refried beans on the stove or in the microwave, making sure they're smooth and spreadable.

Shredded Meat or Ground Beef: Cook or heat up shredded chicken, beef, or ground beef seasoned with Mexican spices (like cumin, chili powder, and garlic) for extra flavor.

Chopped Veggies: Dice tomatoes, onions, and slice lettuce or cabbage thinly for a fresh and crunchy topping.

Guacamole or Avocado: Mash avocado with a bit of lime juice, salt, and pepper for a simple guacamole, or slice it for topping.

3. Assemble the Tostadas

To assemble each tostada, start by spreading a thin layer of refried beans on the crispy tortilla base. Add a layer of your preferred protein, such as shredded chicken or ground beef. Top with shredded lettuce or cabbage, then add a spoonful of diced tomatoes, onions, and any other toppings you like.

Finish with a sprinkle of crumbled queso fresco, a drizzle of Mexican crema, and a dash of hot sauce or salsa. Garnish with fresh cilantro and serve with lime wedges on the side.

4. Serve and Enjoy

Serve the tostadas immediately to maintain the crunchiness of the tortilla. Let everyone customize their own tostadas with additional toppings and sauces for a fun, interactive meal.

Tips for Perfect Tostadas

Use Fresh Corn Tortillas: Fresh, high-quality tortillas make for the best tostadas, as they're sturdy and crisp up nicely.

Avoid Overloading: Tostadas can be a bit messy if overfilled. Add your toppings in layers but keep each layer thin for easier handling.

Serve Immediately: Tostadas are best enjoyed fresh, as the toppings can soften the tortilla if they sit too long.

Experiment with Toppings: Tostadas are a blank canvas, so feel free to experiment with toppings based on your preferences and what you have on hand.

Variations of Tostadas

While this recipe is for a classic tostada, you can customize it with different toppings and flavors:

Seafood Tostadas: Top with ceviche or shrimp for a refreshing and flavorful twist.

Vegetarian Tostadas: Skip the meat and pile on refried beans, guacamole, grilled veggies, and a sprinkle of cheese for a tasty vegetarian option.

Tostadas de Tinga: Make a tinga-style tostada by topping it with shredded chicken cooked in a spicy tomato sauce.

Breakfast Tostadas: Top with scrambled or fried eggs, refried beans, avocado, and a drizzle of hot sauce for breakfast twist.

Serving Suggestions

Tostadas are a complete meal on their own, but they also pair well with other Mexican dishes:

Mexican Rice: Serve a side of Mexican rice to complement the flavors of the tostadas.

Refried Beans or Black Beans: A side of beans adds protein and makes the meal more filling.

Salsa or Hot Sauce: Offer a variety of salsa or hot sauces so everyone can spice their tostadas to their liking.

Aguas Frescas: Fresh fruit drinks like horchata, tamarind, or agua de jamaica are refreshing and balance the savory flavors of the tostadas.

The Cultural Significance of Tostadas

Tostadas are a popular dish across Mexico, enjoyed in different ways depending on the region. Their origins are simple: tostadas were a way to repurpose leftover or slightly stale tortillas by frying them, giving them new life and a crunchy texture. They're often enjoyed as a quick snack or a family meal, and their versatility means they can be topped with ingredients that suit every dish.

Frequently Asked Questions

Q: Can I make tostadas in advance?

You can prepare the tostada bases ahead of time by frying or baking them, then storing them in an airtight container. Assemble with toppings just before serving to keep the tostadas crispy.

Q: Can I use store-bought tostada shells?

Yes, store-bought tostada shells work well if you're short on time. Just make sure to choose ones that are fresh and crispy.

Q: How can I make tostadas healthier?

For a lighter option, bake the tortillas instead of frying. You can also use toppings like grilled veggies, avocado, and lean proteins.

Q: What type of beans should I use?

Refried beans, black beans, or even pinto beans work great as a base for tostadas. Homemade or canned beans are both good options, just make sure they're smooth and spreadable.

Why You'll Love This Tostadas Recipe

This tostadas recipe is easy, customizable, and brings together a variety of delicious flavors and textures. The crispy tortilla base contrasts perfectly with creamy beans, fresh veggies, savory meat, and all the colorful toppings. It's an interactive meal that lets everyone create their own perfect tostada, making it ideal for family meals, casual gatherings, or even quick dinners. Whether you're making classic tostadas with refried beans and cheese or getting creative with toppings like seafood or grilled veggies, these tostadas offer a delicious taste of Mexican cuisine that's sure to become a favorite in your home. Enjoy the crunch, the flavor, and the endless topping possibilities of homemade tostadas!

35

Chiles en Nogada Recipe

Chiles en Nogada is one of Mexico's most iconic and patriotic dishes, celebrated for its vibrant colors and rich flavors. The dish consists of poblano chiles stuffed with a savory-sweet picadillo filling, topped with a creamy walnut sauce (nogada), and garnished with pomegranate seeds and fresh parsley. This unique combination of flavors and colors is said to represent the Mexican flag, making chiles en nogada a popular dish for Mexican Independence Day and other celebrations.

With a balance of sweet, savory, and creamy flavors, chiles en nogada is a gourmet dish that's worth the effort. This recipe provides a step-by-step guide to making authentic chiles en nogada at home.

Ingredients

For the Chiles:

6 large poblano chiles

For the Picadillo Filling:

1 lb. ground beef or pork (or a combination)

1 small onion, finely chopped

2 garlic cloves, minced

1/2 cup of diced tomato

1/2 cup diced apple (such as Gala or Fuji)

1/4 cup diced ripe plantain or banana

1/4 cup diced pear

1/4 cup of raisins

1/4 cup chopped almonds

1/4 tsp of ground cinnamon

1/4 tsp ground cloves

1/4 tsp of ground black pepper

Salt, to taste

1 tbsp vegetable oil

For the Nogada (Walnut Sauce):

1 cup of walnuts, soaked in hot water for at least 1 hour, then drained

1/2 cup milk or heavy cream

4 oz cream cheese (optional, for a thicker sauce)

1 tbsp sugar (adjust to taste)

1/4 tsp of ground cinnamon

Salt, to taste

For Garnish:

1/2 cup pomegranate seeds

Fresh parsley leaves, chopped

Step-by-Step Instructions

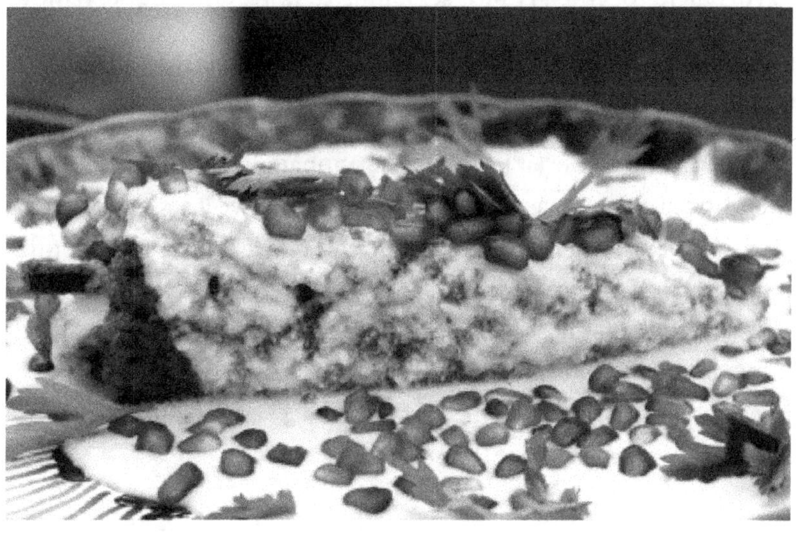

1. ROAST AND PEEL THE Poblanos

Start by roasting the poblano chiles over an open flame, on a gas stove, or in a hot skillet until the skin is evenly charred. Place the chiles in a plastic or paper bag and let them steam for about 10 minutes. This makes it easier to peel the skin off.

Once cooled, gently peel off the charred skin. Be careful not to tear the chile. Make a small slit down the side of each chile and carefully remove the seeds and veins. Set the chiles aside to prepare the filling.

2. Make the Picadillo Filling

In a large skillet, heat the vegetable oil over medium heat. Add the chopped onion and garlic and cook until they're soft and translucent. Add the ground meat and cook until browned, breaking it up with a spoon as it cooks.

Stir in the diced tomato, apple, plantain, pear, raisins, almonds, cinnamon, cloves, black pepper, and salt. Let the mixture simmer for 10-15 minutes, stirring occasionally, until the fruit softens and the flavors meld together. Adjust seasoning to taste. Once done, remove the skillet from heat and let the filling cool slightly.

3. Prepare the Walnut Sauce (Nogada)

In a blender, combine the soaked and drained walnuts, milk (or cream), cream cheese (if using), sugar, cinnamon, and a pinch of salt. Blend until smooth and creamy. Adjust the sweetness and salt to taste. The sauce should be thick but pourable, so add a bit more milk if needed to achieve the desired consistency.

4. Stuff the Chiles

Carefully stuff each poblano chile with the picadillo filling, being careful not to overfill or tear the chile. Use a spoon to gently pack the filling into the chile through the slit.

5. Plate and Serve

Place the stuffed chiles on a serving platter or individual plates. Generously spoon the walnut sauce over each chile, covering the top.

Sprinkle with pomegranate seeds and fresh parsley for a burst of color.

Serve the chiles en nogada at room temperature for the best flavor, though they can also be served slightly warm.

Tips for Perfect Chiles en Nogada

Roast the Poblanos Well: Roasting and peeling the poblano chiles is essential for a smooth texture and smoky flavor. Be careful not to tear the chiles when peeling or stuffing.

Soak the Walnuts: Soaking the walnuts helps remove any bitterness and creates a smoother sauce.

Adjust the Sweetness: The walnut sauce should have a hint of sweetness to balance the savory filling. Adjust the sugar in the sauce to taste.

Serve at Room Temperature: Chiles en nogada are traditionally served at room temperature, allowing the flavors to shine without the sauce melting off.

Variations of Chiles en Nogada

While this recipe is traditional, there are ways to adapt it based on your taste or dietary preferences:

Vegetarian Chiles en Nogada: Replace the meat with finely chopped mushrooms, tofu, or additional vegetables like zucchini for a vegetarian filling.

Vegan Chiles en Nogada: Use a dairy-free cream substitute for the nogada and skip the cream cheese for a vegan option.

Chicken Chiles en Nogada: Substitute ground pork or beef with shredded chicken for a lighter filling.

Spicy Chiles en Nogada: For a spicier version, add a bit of chopped jalapeño or serrano pepper to the picadillo filling.

Serving Suggestions

Chiles en nogada is often enjoyed as a complete meal, but here are some ideas for pairing it with other dishes:

Mexican Rice: A side of Mexican rice complements the flavors and adds to the meal.

Fresh Salad: A simple green salad with a lime vinaigrette pair well and balances the richness of the dish.

Mexican Beer or Wine: A crisp Mexican beer or a light white wine, like a Sauvignon Blanc, pairs wonderfully with the dish.

The History of Chiles en Nogada

Chiles en nogada has a rich cultural significance in Mexican cuisine, especially in the state of Puebla where it originated. The dish was reportedly created by Augustinian nuns in Puebla to celebrate the independence of Mexico. The green poblano chiles, white walnut sauce, and red pomegranate seeds are said to represent the colors of the Mexican flag. Chiles en nogada is often enjoyed during patriotic holidays, especially around Mexican Independence Day in September, symbolizing Mexican pride and culinary heritage.

Frequently Asked Questions

Q: Can I make chiles en nogada in advance?

Yes, you can make the picadillo filling and walnut sauce a day in advance. Store the filling and sauce separately in the refrigerator, and stuff the chiles just before serving.

Q: Can I freeze chiles en nogada?

It's best to enjoy chiles en nogada fresh, as freezing can affect the texture of the sauce. However, you can freeze the picadillo filling separately and make the sauce fresh when ready to serve.

Q: What is the best type of apple to use for chiles en nogada?

A sweet, firm apple like Gala, Fuji, or Golden Delicious works well in the picadillo filling, adding a mild sweetness that complements the other flavors.

Q: Do I have to use cream cheese in the walnut sauce?

Cream cheese is optional and adds thickness to the sauce, but you can omit it if you prefer a lighter, more traditional nogada sauce.

Why You'll Love This Chiles en Nogada Recipe

This chiles en nogada recipe is an exquisite combination of flavors, textures, and colors that truly capture the essence of Mexican cuisine. With the slightly smoky poblano chiles, sweet-savory picadillo filling, creamy walnut sauce, and bursts of fresh pomegranate, each bite has a delicious balance of contrasting flavors and textures. Chiles en nogada is a dish that celebrates tradition, culture, and culinary artistry. Whether you're making it for a special occasion or simply to enjoy the flavors of Mexico, this recipe offers an authentic and memorable experience that's sure to impress. Enjoy this taste of Mexican heritage and treat yourself to the beautiful and delicious creation that is chiles en nogada!

36

Elote Recipe

E lote, also known as Mexican street corn, is a popular Mexican snack that combines the sweetness of grilled corn with creamy, tangy, and spicy flavors. Traditionally served on the cob and smothered in mayonnaise, cotija cheese, lime, and chili powder, elote is a delicious, easy-to-make treat that's perfect for barbecues, family gatherings, or even a quick snack. This dish is easy to customize, making it a hit with everyone who tries it!

Here's a recipe that will guide you through making authentic elote at home, along with tips for grilling, seasoning, and adding toppings to make it your own.

Ingredients

4 ears of corn, husked

1/4 cup of mayonnaise

1/4 cup Mexican crema or sour cream

1/2 cup crumbled cotija cheese (or feta as a substitute)

1 lime, cut into wedges

1 tbsp chili powder or Tajín seasoning (adjust to taste)

Fresh cilantro, chopped (for garnish, optional)

Optional Toppings:

Hot sauce (such as Valentina or Cholula)

Extra lime wedges

Smoked paprika for added smokiness

Step-by-Step Instructions

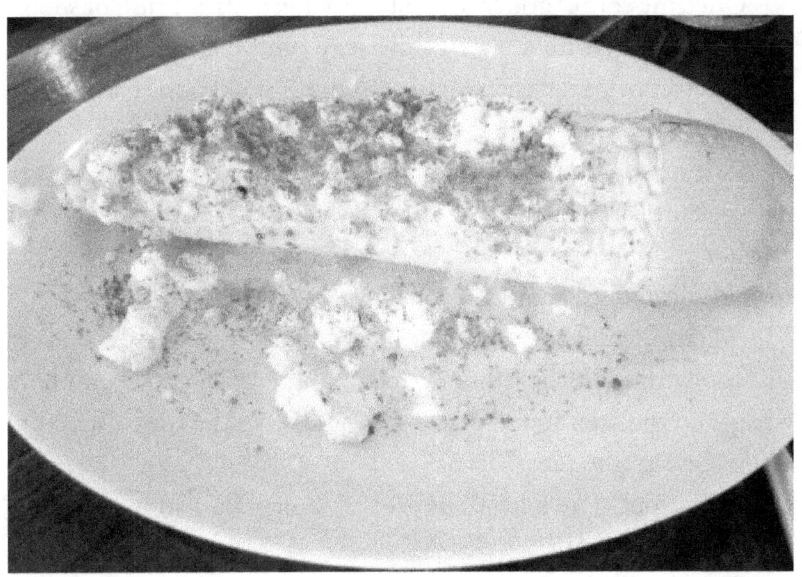

1. PREHEAT THE GRILL

Preheat your grill to medium-high heat (about 400°F or 200°C). If you don't have a grill, you can also cook the corn under the broiler in your oven or on a stovetop grill pan.

2. Grill the Corn

Place the ears of corn directly on the grill and cook, turning occasionally, until they are tender and slightly charred on all sides, about 8-10 minutes. The charred spots add flavor and help the toppings adhere to the corn.

If using a broiler or stovetop pan, cook the corn until charred, turning every few minutes for even cooking.

3. Prepare the Toppings

In a small bowl, mix the mayonnaise and Mexican crema (or sour cream) until smooth. Set aside. Arrange the crumbled cotija cheese, chili powder, and lime wedges within reach so you can quickly assemble the elotes once the corn is cooked.

4. Coat the Corn

Once the corn is grilled and slightly cooled, use a brush or spoon to coat each ear with a layer of the mayo and crema mixture. This creamy layer helps the cheese and seasonings stick to the corn.

5. Add the Cheese and Seasonings

Roll or sprinkle the coated corn with crumbled cotija cheese, making sure it sticks to the creamy layer. Then, sprinkle with chili powder or Tajín to your desired level of spice. For extra flavor, add a sprinkle of smoked paprika if you like.

6. Garnish and Serve

Top with fresh cilantro if desired and serve the elotes with lime wedges on the side. Squeeze fresh lime juice over the corn just before eating for a bright, tangy flavor.

Enjoy your elote hot off the grill, with napkins handy—it's a deliciously messy treat!

Tips for Perfect Elote

Use Fresh Corn: Fresh, sweet corn is ideal for elote, as its natural sugars caramelize on the grill, enhancing the flavor.

Customize the Spice: If you prefer less spice, use a milder chili powder or a sprinkle of smoked paprika for flavor without the heat.

Use Quality Cheese: Cotija cheese is traditional and provides a salty, crumbly texture. If you can't find cotija, feta cheese is a good substitute.

Serve Immediately: Elote is best enjoyed fresh off the grill while still warm and creamy.

Variations of Elote

While the classic recipe is delicious as is, there are plenty of ways to customize your elote:

Elote with Hot Sauce: Drizzle your favorite hot sauce over the corn for extra spice.

Elote en Vaso: Also known as esquites, this variation serves the corn off the cob in a cup, mixed with all the toppings for easier eating.

Cheesy Elote: Add a sprinkle of grated Parmesan or shredded cheese along with the cotija for extra cheesiness.

Garlic Elote: Mix a bit of minced garlic into the mayo-crema mixture for an added savory kick.

Serving Suggestions

Elote is a versatile side that pairs well with other Mexican dishes and grilled foods:

Tacos: Serve elote alongside grilled tacos or street-style carne asada tacos for a complete Mexican-inspired meal.

Grilled Meats: Pair with grilled chicken, steak, or ribs for a hearty barbecue spread.

Mexican Rice: A side of Mexican rice or refried beans makes a filling and flavorful addition.

Fresh Salad: Balance the richness of elote with a light salad, such as a cucumber and avocado salad with lime dressing.

The Cultural Significance of Elote

Elote is a staple street food in Mexico, enjoyed as a snack or quick meal by people of all ages. Vendors can often be found selling elotes on city streets, especially in the evening, when the aroma of grilled corn fills the air. With its roots in Mesoamerican cuisine, corn has long been a central part of Mexican culture and cuisine. The word "elote" comes from the Nahuatl word "elotl," meaning "tender cob." Today, elote remains a beloved comfort food that's simple yet full of flavor.

Frequently Asked Questions

Q: Can I make elote in advance?

Elote is best enjoyed fresh, but you can grill the corn ahead of time and reheat it on the grill just before serving. Wait until adding the mayo, cheese, and toppings until right before serving.

Q: Can I use frozen corn?

Yes, you can use frozen corn if fresh isn't available. Thaw the corn, then grill or roast it as fresh corn. While the flavor won't be quite the same as fresh corn, it's still delicious.

Q: What's the difference between elote and esquites?

Elote is served on the cob, while esquites is the off-the-cob version, where the corn is mixed with all the toppings in a cup or bowl for easier eating.

Q: Can I make Elote vegan?

Yes! Use vegan mayonnaise and a plant-based cheese alternative to make vegan elote. You can also skip the crema and add extra lime juice for tanginess.

Why You'll Love This Elote Recipe

This elote recipe combines the smoky sweetness of grilled corn with a creamy, tangy topping that's hard to resist. The layers of flavor from the cotija cheese, chili powder, and fresh lime juice create a balanced bite that's both rich and refreshing. With simple preparation and endless topping possibilities, elote is a crowd-pleasing addition to any meal, whether as a side, snack, or main attraction. Perfect for summer gatherings, outdoor barbecues, or even a cozy indoor meal, elote brings authentic Mexican street food flavor right to your home. Enjoy the taste, tradition, and vibrant flavor of this classic Mexican dish!

37

Mole Recipe

M ole is one of Mexico's most beloved sauces, known for its deep, rich, and complex flavors. Often made with a combination of chiles, spices, nuts, seeds, chocolate, and dried fruits, mole is a versatile sauce that varies by region. The word "mole" is derived from the Nahuatl word mōlli, meaning "sauce" or "concoction." While there are many types of mole, this recipe focuses on the classic mole poblano, which is traditionally served with chicken or turkey.

Making mole from scratch can take time, but the result is a flavorful sauce with a perfect balance of smoky, sweet, spicy, and earthy notes. Here's a step-by-step guide to making an authentic mole poblano that will bring the taste of Mexico to your kitchen.

Ingredients

For the Sauce:

4 dried ancho chiles, stemmed and seeded

4 dried guajillo chiles, stemmed and seeded

2 dried pasilla chiles, stemmed and seeded

1/4 cup vegetable oil or lard (for frying)

1/2 cup almonds or peanuts

1/4 cup of pumpkin seeds (pepitas)

1/4 cup of sesame seeds

1/2 cup of raisins

1 small corn tortilla, torn into pieces

2 slices of stale bread or 1 bolillo roll, torn into pieces

1 large onion, chopped

4 garlic cloves

2 tomatoes, chopped

1 plantain or ripe banana, sliced

1 cinnamon stick or 1/2 tsp ground cinnamon

1/4 tsp ground cloves

1/4 tsp ground allspice

1 tsp dried Mexican oregano

Salt and black pepper, to taste

1/4 cup Mexican chocolate or bittersweet chocolate, chopped

For Assembly:

4-6 pieces of chicken (thighs, drumsticks, or breasts)

Salt, to taste

Fresh cilantro for garnish (optional)

Sesame seeds for garnish

Step-by-Step Instructions

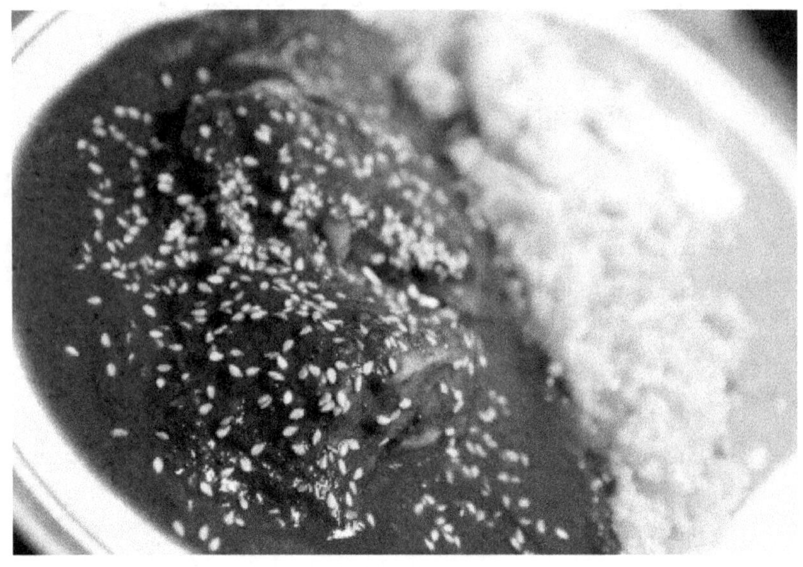

1. TOAST AND SOAK THE Chiles

In a dry skillet over medium heat, toast the ancho, guajillo, and pasilla chiles until they become fragrant, for about 1-2 minutes. Be careful not to burn them, as this can make the mole bitter.

Transfer the toasted chiles to a bowl, cover them with hot water, and let them soak for about 15-20 minutes, or until softened. Once softened, remove the chiles from the water and set aside. Reserve the soaking water.

2. Fry the Ingredients

In a large skillet, heat the vegetable oil or lard over medium heat. Working in batches, fry the almonds, pumpkin seeds, sesame seeds, and raisins until golden and fragrant. The raisins will puff up, and the seeds will lightly brown. Remove each ingredient from the skillet and set aside.

In the same skillet, add the tortilla and bread pieces, frying until golden brown. Remove from the skillet and set aside.

Next, add the chopped onion, garlic cloves, tomatoes, and sliced plantain or banana to the skillet. Sauté until the vegetables are softened and caramelized, about 5-7 minutes.

3. Blend the Mole Paste

In a blender, combine the softened chiles, fried almonds, pumpkin seeds, sesame seeds, raisins, tortilla, bread, onion, garlic, tomatoes, and plantain. Add the cinnamon stick (or ground cinnamon), ground cloves, allspice, oregano, and a pinch of salt and pepper. Blend the ingredients until smooth, adding the reserved chile soaking water a little at a time to create a thick paste.

Depending on the size of your blender, you may need to blend in batches.

4. Simmer the Mole Sauce

Transfer the mole paste to a large pot over medium heat. Stirring constantly, cook the paste for about 10 minutes, allowing it to thicken and deepen in flavor.

Add 4 cups of chicken broth (or water if preferred) and bring to a simmer. Reduce the heat to low and let the mole simmer for about 30-45 minutes, stirring occasionally. Add more broth as needed to reach your desired consistency; mole should be thick but pourable.

5. Add the Chocolate

Add the Mexican chocolate or bittersweet chocolate to the mole and stir until melted and well incorporated. Taste the sauce and adjust the seasoning with salt, pepper, or additional spices if needed. The chocolate adds richness and a hint of sweetness that balances the smoky and spicy flavors of the mole.

6. Cook the Chicken

While the mole simmers, season the chicken pieces with salt. In a separate pot, boil the chicken in water until fully cooked, for about 20-30 minutes. Once cooked, drain the chicken pieces.

7. Serve the Mole

Place the cooked chicken pieces on a serving platter and generously spoon the mole sauce over the top. Garnish with fresh cilantro and a sprinkle of sesame seeds for extra flavor and texture.

Serve your mole with warm corn tortillas and a side of Mexican rice for a traditional meal.

Tips for Perfect Mole

Toast the Ingredients Well: Toasting the chiles, nuts, seeds, and bread is key to unlocking their flavors and adding depth to the mole.

Use Mexican Chocolate: Mexican chocolate is traditional in mole poblano. If unavailable, bittersweet chocolate works well.

Adjust Consistency: Mole should be thick but smooth and pourable. Adjust the consistency by adding more broth or water as needed.

Patience is Key: Mole is best when cooked low and slow, allowing the flavors to meld together over time.

Variations of Mole

Mole is incredibly versatile and varies greatly across different regions of Mexico. Some popular variations include:

Mole Verde: This green mole uses ingredients like tomatillos, green chiles, fresh herbs, and pumpkin seeds. It has a lighter, tangier flavor.

Mole Amarillo: A yellow mole that's popular in Oaxaca, made with yellow chiles, masa, and vegetables, giving it a unique color and taste.

Mole Negro: A darker mole that includes more chocolate and additional ingredients like hoja santa, making it one of the richest and most complex moles.

Serving Suggestions

Mole poblano is typically served with sides that complement its rich flavors:

Mexican Rice: A side of fluffy Mexican rice is perfect for soaking up the mole sauce.

Warm Corn Tortillas: Tortillas are essential for scooping up every last bit of mole.

Black Beans: A side of black beans adds protein and balances the richness of the mole.

The History of Mole

Mole has a deep cultural significance in Mexico, with roots in both pre-Hispanic and colonial influences. The sauce is believed to have originated in the convents of Puebla and Oaxaca, where nuns combined indigenous ingredients like chiles and chocolate with spices brought by Spanish colonists. Mole is often associated with celebrations, weddings, and holidays, where it's served as a special meal for gatherings. Today, mole remains a symbol of Mexican culinary heritage and regional pride.

Frequently Asked Questions

Q: Can I make mole in advance?

Yes, mole is often better the next day, as the flavors continue to develop. Store it in the refrigerator for up to 5 days. Reheat on the stove, adding a bit of water or broth if it thickens.

Q: Can I freeze mole?

Absolutely! Mole freezes well and can be stored in a freezer-safe container for up to 3 months. Thaw in the refrigerator and reheat on the stove.

Q: Is mole spicy?

Mole has a mild to moderate spice level, depending on the types and quantities of chiles used. You can adjust the heat by adding more or fewer chiles to suit your taste.

Q: Can I use store-bought mole paste?

Yes, store-bought mole paste is a convenient alternative. Simply rehydrate it with chicken broth and add a bit of chocolate or extra spices to enhance the flavor.

Why You'll Love This Mole Recipe

This mole recipe brings out the authentic flavors of Mexico with its rich, complex sauce that balances smoky, spicy, sweet, and earthy notes. Mole is a labor of love, but the time spent toasting, blending, and simmering each ingredient results in a sauce that's truly unforgettable. Perfect for special occasions or as a delicious homemade treat, this mole poblano pairs beautifully with chicken, turkey, or even roasted vegetables. Enjoy the layers of flavor and the cultural heritage that mole represents in every bite. Mole is more than just a sauce—it's a celebration of Mexican cuisine, history, and tradition.

38

Quesadillas Recipe

Quesadillas are a beloved Mexican dish featuring melted cheese between two tortillas, lightly grilled until golden and crispy. While the classic version is simply cheese, quesadillas can be customized with a variety of fillings—from sautéed vegetables and shredded chicken to mushrooms and beans. They're quick, easy to make, and perfect for any meal, whether it's breakfast, lunch, dinner, or even a snack.

This recipe walks you through making traditional cheese quesadillas, along with ideas for tasty fillings and tips for achieving that perfect crispy texture.

Ingredients

4 large flour or corn tortillas

1 1/2 cups of shredded cheese (such as Oaxaca, Monterey Jack, or cheddar)

1 tbsp vegetable oil or butter

Optional Fillings:

1/2 cup cooked shredded chicken or beef

1/2 cup sautéed bell peppers and onions

1/4 cup of refried beans

1/4 cup of diced tomatoes

Fresh jalapeño slices for a spicy kick

Fresh spinach or mushrooms

Toppings and Dips:

Fresh salsa or pico de gallo

Guacamole

Sour cream or Mexican crema

Fresh cilantro

Step-by-Step Instructions

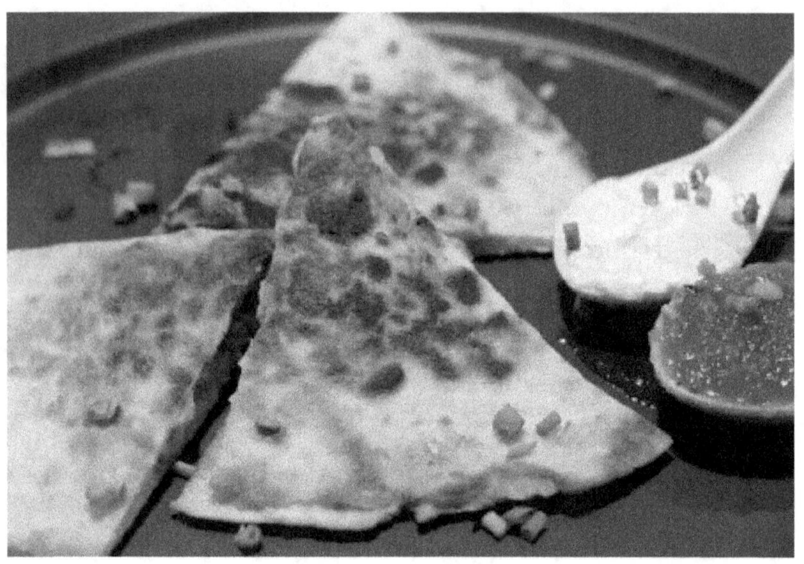

1. PREPARE YOUR FILLING Ingredients

If you're using additional fillings, prepare them in advance. For example, cook and shred the chicken or beef, sauté the vegetables, or warm up refried beans. This way, everything is ready to add to your quesadilla as soon as you start cooking.

2. Heat the Skillet

Place a large skillet or griddle over medium heat. Add a small amount of vegetable oil or butter to lightly coat the pan; this helps create a golden, crispy texture on the tortilla.

3. Assemble the Quesadilla

Lay one tortilla flat in the skillet and sprinkle an even layer of cheese on one half of the tortilla, leaving a little space around the edges. Add any additional fillings you like on top of the cheese, being careful not to overfill.

Once the fillings are added, fold the tortilla in half to cover the cheese and fillings. This method allows for easier flipping and an evenly melted filling.

4. Cook the Quesadilla

Cook the quesadilla for about 2-3 minutes on each side, or until the tortilla is golden brown and crispy, and the cheese is melted. Use a spatula to press down gently on the quesadilla to help it cook evenly.

For extra-large quesadillas, you can cook them open-faced by adding the second tortilla on top or cook with both tortillas flat and slice into quarters after cooking.

5. Repeat with Remaining Tortillas

Repeat the process with the remaining tortillas, adding a little more oil or butter if needed.

6. Slice and Serve

Transfer the cooked quesadilla to a cutting board and let it cool slightly. Slice it into wedges and serve with your choice of toppings and dips, like salsa, guacamole, and sour cream.

Enjoy your quesadilla while it's still warm, as this is when it's at its crispiest and cheesiest.

Tips for Perfect Quesadillas

Choose the Right Cheese: Mexican cheeses like Oaxaca or queso asadero melt beautifully and have a mild, creamy flavor. Cheddar, Monterey Jack, and Mozzarella are also excellent options.

Don't Overfill: Too many fillings can make it difficult to cook the quesadilla evenly and may cause it to fall apart. Keep the filling light and even.

Cook on Medium Heat: Cooking over medium heat allows the cheese to melt without burning the tortilla.

Use Butter or Oil Sparingly: A light coating of butter or oil gives a crispy texture without making the quesadilla too greasy.

Variations of Quesadillas

While a classic cheese quesadilla is always delicious, there are some fun variations to try:

Chicken Quesadilla: Add shredded chicken seasoned with spices like cumin, chili powder, and garlic for a hearty filling.

Vegetable Quesadilla: Use sautéed bell peppers, onions, mushrooms, and spinach for a healthy and flavorful veggie version.

Breakfast Quesadilla: Add scrambled eggs, cheese, and cooked breakfast sausage or bacon for a tasty breakfast option.

BBQ Quesadilla: Mix in shredded BBQ chicken or pulled pork with cheese for a sweet and savory twist.

Serving Suggestions

Quesadillas are versatile and pair well with a variety of Mexican-inspired sides and toppings:

Salsa or Pico de Gallo: Fresh salsa adds brightness and flavor to each bite.

Guacamole: Creamy guacamole is a perfect pairing with the cheesy quesadilla.

Mexican Rice: Serve a side of Mexican rice for a filling, well-rounded meal.

Refried Beans: A side of refried beans complements the flavors and adds extra protein.

The Origins of Quesadillas

Quesadillas have been enjoyed in Mexico for centuries and originally come from the region of Oaxaca. In the early days, they were typically made with corn tortillas and simple fillings like cheese or squash blossoms, called flor de calabaza. As the dish spread and evolved, flour tortillas became popular in northern Mexico and the United States. Today, quesadillas are enjoyed in a variety of forms, from street food stalls to home kitchens, as a beloved Mexican comfort food.

Frequently Asked Questions

Q: Can I use corn tortillas instead of flour tortillas?

Absolutely! Corn tortillas are traditional in many regions of Mexico and add a distinct flavor. Just be aware that corn tortillas are smaller and less pliable, so they're best for single-layer quesadillas.

Q: Can I make quesadillas ahead of time?

Quesadillas are best enjoyed fresh, but you can prep the fillings in advance. If you do need to make them ahead, cook the quesadillas and reheat them in a hot skillet to restore their crispiness.

Q: How can I make quesadillas healthier?

Use whole wheat tortillas, add plenty of veggies, and go light on the cheese for a healthier version. You can also use low-fat cheese if preferred.

Q: What's the best way to reheat a quesadilla?

Reheat quesadillas in a skillet or on a griddle over medium heat to restore their crispy texture. Avoid the microwave, as it can make the tortillas soggy.

Why You'll Love This Quesadillas Recipe

This Quesadilla recipe is easy, adaptable, and endlessly satisfying. With its crispy tortilla, melty cheese, and flavorful fillings, each bite is packed with texture and taste. Quesadillas are perfect for any occasion, whether you're whipping up a quick snack, feeding a crowd, or making a fun and interactive meal with friends or family. Customize them with your favorite ingredients, serve them with fresh toppings, and enjoy a delicious, homemade taste of Mexico. Quesadillas are simple yet full of flavor, making them a go-to recipe for any day of the week!

39

Agua Fresca Recipe

Agua fresca, meaning "fresh water" in Spanish, is a traditional Mexican beverage made by blending fresh fruits, water, and a touch of sweetener for a naturally refreshing drink. It's perfect for cooling off on hot days, serving at gatherings, or simply as a delicious alternative to sugary sodas. With its fresh, vibrant flavor, agua fresca is both hydrating and full of natural goodness.

This basic agua fresca recipe is versatile, allowing you to use any fresh fruit you like. From classic flavors like watermelon, cucumber, and cantaloupe to more adventurous combinations, you can make endless varieties of this beloved drink.

Ingredients

4 cups of fresh fruit of choice (such as watermelon, cantaloupe, mango, pineapple, or strawberries)

4 cups of cold water, divided

1-2 tbsp sugar or agave syrup (adjust to taste)

Juice of 1 lime (optional, for added brightness)

Ice cubes, for serving

Optional Garnishes:

Fresh mint leaves

Lime wedges

Cucumber slices

Step-by-Step Instructions

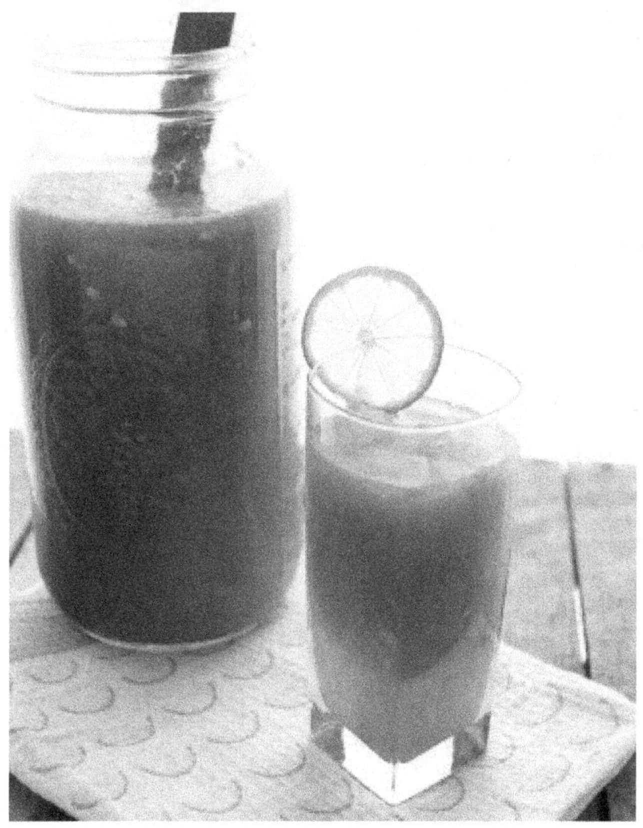

1. PREPARE THE FRUIT

If necessary, peel and remove any seeds from the fruit you're using. Cut it into chunks that will be easy to blend. For melons, mangoes, and pineapples, this will also help release their natural juices and make the blending process easier.

2. Blend the Fruit

Place the fruit chunks in a blender along with 2 cups of cold water. Blend until the mixture is smooth. If you prefer a pulpier drink, you can blend it for a shorter time.

3. Strain the Mixture (Optional)

If you like a smooth agua fresca, pour the blended fruit mixture through a fine-mesh strainer into a large pitcher. Use a spoon to press the pulp and extract as much juice as possible. This step is optional; if you enjoy pulp, you can skip straining.

4. Add Sweetener and Water

Add the remaining 2 cups of water to the pitcher and stir in sugar or agave syrup to taste. If desired, squeeze in the juice for 1 lime for a hint of acidity and brightness.

5. Chill and Serve

Place the pitcher in the refrigerator to chill for at least 30 minutes. When ready to serve, pour the agua fresca over ice cubes in individual glasses.

Garnish with fresh mint leaves, a lime wedge, or cucumber slices for extra flair. Enjoy your refreshing agua fresca on a hot day or with your favorite Mexican dishes!

Tips for Perfect Agua Fresca

Adjust the Sweetness: Some fruits, like watermelon and mango, are naturally sweet and may not need extra sugar. Taste the blended mixture before adding sweetener to avoid making it too sugary.

Use Cold Water: Starting with cold water makes for an instantly refreshing drink, especially if you don't have time to chill it in the fridge.

Experiment with Flavors: Try mixing different fruits to create unique flavors, such as pineapple-mint, mango-cucumber, or strawberry-watermelon.

Add Fresh Herbs: Fresh herbs like mint, basil, or cilantro add an interesting layer of flavor and pair well with fruits like watermelon, cucumber, and pineapple.

Popular Agua Fresca Flavor Ideas

While you can use almost any fruit, here are some popular agua fresca flavors to try:

Watermelon Agua Fresca: A classic choice, made simply with watermelon, lime, and a touch of sugar.

Cucumber Lime Agua Fresca: Refreshing and light, perfect for hot days. Add fresh mint or basil for extra flavor.

Mango Agua Fresca: Blend fresh mango with lime juice and a pinch of salt for a tropical twist.

Pineapple Agua Fresca: Sweet and slightly tangy, pineapple agua fresca pairs well with mint or a splash of coconut water.

Strawberry Agua Fresca: Sweet and vibrant, this version tastes delicious with a hint of lime or a few fresh basil leaves.

Serving Suggestions

Agua fresca is a versatile drink that pairs well with a variety of Mexican dishes and snacks:

Tacos: Serve agua fresca alongside tacos, burritos, or enchiladas for a refreshing contrast to spicy flavors.

Grilled Foods: The cool, fruity taste of agua fresca complements grilled meats, seafood, and veggies perfectly.

Light Appetizers: Agua fresca pairs well with appetizers like chips and guacamole, salsa, and ceviche.

Desserts: Serve with Mexican desserts like churros or tres leches cake for a sweet, refreshing drink to balance the richness of dessert.

The Origins of Agua Fresca

Agua fresca has a long history in Mexico and Latin America, where fresh, local fruits are abundant. Street vendors in Mexico often sell agua fresca by the cup, especially in busy markets, plazas, and during festivals. This traditional drink is cherished for its simple preparation and fresh ingredients, making it a delicious way to stay hydrated in hot weather.

Today, agua fresca has become popular worldwide, enjoyed for its refreshing qualities and endless flavor possibilities. It's also a healthy choice, as it's made with real fruit and typically contains far less sugar than commercial sodas.

Frequently Asked Questions

Q: Can I make agua fresca in advance?

Yes, agua fresca can be made a day in advance. Store it in the refrigerator in a covered pitcher and stir before serving, as the fruit pulp may settle at the bottom.

Q: Can I use frozen fruit?

Yes, frozen fruit works well, especially for tropical fruits like mango and pineapple. It also makes the drink extra cold, reducing the need for ice.

Q: Can I make agua fresca without added sugar?

Definitely! If the fruit is naturally sweet, you may not need added sugar. You can also use a natural sweetener like honey or agave syrup instead.

Q: What can I do with the leftover fruit pulp?

The leftover fruit pulp can be added to smoothies, used in baked goods, or blended with yogurt for a nutritious snack.

Why You'll Love This Agua Fresca Recipe

This agua fresca recipe is simple, refreshing, and packed with natural fruit flavor. It's a healthy, low-sugar drink that you can enjoy at any time of the day, whether as a cooling beverage or alongside a meal. With endless fruit combinations and a touch of lime for brightness, every sip is bursting with freshness. Perfect for summer picnics, barbecues, and family gatherings, agua fresca is a delicious way to stay hydrated and enjoy the taste of fresh fruit. Give this recipe a try and savor the authentic taste of Mexico's most refreshing drink!

40

Ceviche Recipe

Ceviche is a beloved Latin American dish made with fresh seafood that's "cooked" in citrus juice, typically lime or lemon, and mixed with fresh vegetables and herbs. The acidity of the citrus transforms the texture of the fish, giving it a tender yet firm bite. This refreshing dish is popular along coastal regions and is enjoyed as an appetizer or light meal, especially during warm weather.

While there are many variations, this recipe will guide you through making a classic fish ceviche with simple, fresh ingredients. It's easy to make and incredibly satisfying, with a balance of tangy, spicy, and herbaceous flavors.

Ingredients

1 lb. fresh white fish, such as sea bass, tilapia, snapper, or halibut, diced into small cubes

1 cup fresh lime juice (about 8-10 limes)

1/2 cup fresh lemon juice (optional, for added flavor)

1/2 red onion, finely diced

1 small cucumber, diced (optional)

1/2 cup of diced tomato

1 small jalapeño or serrano pepper, finely diced (remove seeds for less heat)

1/2 cup fresh cilantro, chopped

Salt, to taste

Freshly ground black pepper, to taste

Optional Additions:

1 avocado, diced (for creaminess)

1/2 cup diced mango or pineapple (for a tropical touch)

Extra lime wedges for serving

Step-by-Step Instructions

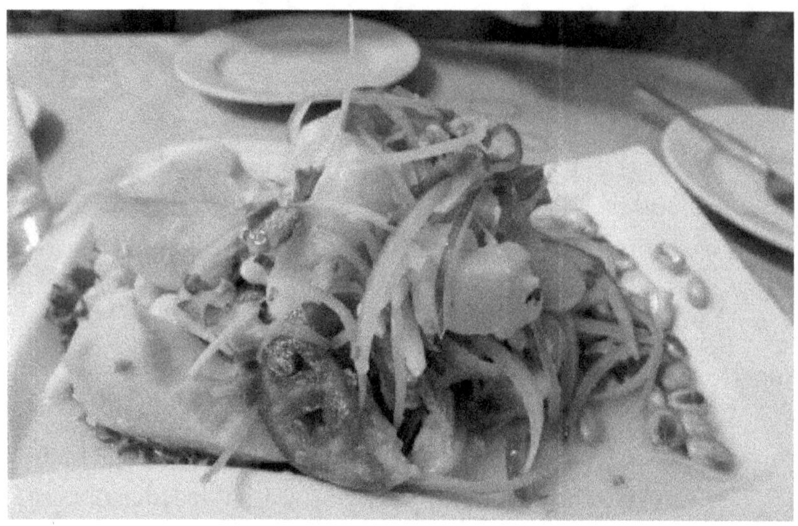

1. PREPARE THE FISH

Make sure your fish is fresh, as ceviche relies on raw seafood that's "cooked" by the citrus juice. Using a sharp knife, dice the fish into small, uniform cubes for even "cooking." Place the diced fish in a glass or ceramic bowl (avoid metal as it can affect the flavor).

2. Marinate the Fish in Citrus

Pour the lime juice (and lemon juice, if using) over the fish, making sure it's fully submerged in the citrus juice. Cover the bowl with plastic wrap and refrigerate for 15-30 minutes, stirring occasionally. The fish will gradually turn opaque as it "cooks" in the acidic juice. For a more tender texture, marinate for up to 1 hour, but avoid over-marinating to keep the fish from becoming too firm.

3. Add Vegetables and Seasonings

Once the fish is "cooked" to your liking, drain some of the excess citrus juice, leaving just enough to keep it moist. Add the red onion, cucumber, tomato, jalapeño, and chopped cilantro. Stir to combine. Season the ceviche with salt and pepper to taste, adjusting as needed.

4. Serve and Garnish

Gently fold in any optional ingredients, such as avocado or diced tropical fruit, for extra flavor and texture. Transfer the ceviche to a serving dish or individual bowls and garnish with extra cilantro, lime wedges, or a sprinkle of additional diced jalapeño for a spicier kick.

Serve the ceviche chilled with tortilla chips, tostadas, or saltine crackers for added crunch.

Tips for Perfect Ceviche

Choose Fresh, High-Quality Fish: Freshness is essential for ceviche, as it's the main ingredient. Buy from a trusted source and look for firm, bright fish.

Use Plenty of Lime Juice: The citrus juice not only adds flavor but also "cooks" the fish, so be sure to use enough to submerge the fish.

Adjust Marinating Time: Different types of fish vary in texture, so adjust the marinating time based on the fish and your preference.

Add Veggies Just Before Serving: For maximum freshness, add vegetables like onions, cucumbers, and tomatoes just before serving.

Variations of Ceviche

While classic fish ceviche is delicious on its own, you can get creative with additional ingredients:

Shrimp Ceviche: Substitute shrimp for fish or use a combination of both. Shrimp ceviche is popular and slightly sweeter.

Mixed Seafood Ceviche: Add scallops, squid, or octopus along with the fish for a more complex flavor and texture.

Fruit-Infused Ceviche: Add diced mango, pineapple, or even orange segments for a tropical touch that pairs well with the acidity of the lime.

Mexican Ceviche: Add diced radishes, a splash of clamato juice, or sprinkle of Tajín for a Mexican twist.

Serving Suggestions

Ceviche is incredibly versatile and can be served in different ways:

Tostadas: Serve the ceviche on top of crispy tostadas for a satisfying crunch.

Tortilla Chips: Scoop up the ceviche with tortilla chips for an easy, crowd-pleasing appetizer.

Crispy Lettuce Cups: For a low-carb option, serve the ceviche in romaine or butter lettuce cups.

Avocado Halves: Scoop ceviche into halved avocados for a beautiful presentation and creamy bite.

The Origins of Ceviche

Ceviche has roots in coastal regions of Latin America, with many countries claiming their own unique versions. It's believed to have originated in Peru, where it's a national dish, but variations of ceviche are also popular in Mexico, Ecuador, and other Latin American countries. Each region uses local ingredients to create distinctive flavors and textures, and ceviche is celebrated as a refreshing, naturally flavorful dish.

Frequently Asked Questions

Q: Can I make ceviche in advance?

Ceviche is best enjoyed fresh, but you can prepare the fish and marinate it up to an hour ahead. For the freshest taste, add the vegetables and seasoning just before serving.

Q: How long does ceviche keep?

Ceviche should be consumed the same day it's made, as the fish will continue to "cook" in the citrus and may become tough if left for too long. Leftovers can be stored in the refrigerator for up to 1 day but may lose texture.

Q: Can I use frozen fish?

Yes, you can use previously frozen fish but ensure it's of high quality and completely thawed. Freezing may alter the texture slightly, but it's a safe option if fresh fish isn't available.

Q: Is ceviche safe to eat?

When prepared properly with fresh, high-quality fish and acidic citrus juice, ceviche is generally safe to eat. However, pregnant individuals or those with compromised immune systems may want to consult a doctor before consuming raw seafood.

Why You'll Love This Ceviche Recipe

This ceviche recipe is light, zesty, and full of fresh flavors, making it a perfect dish for warm days or anytime you crave something vibrant and refreshing. The combination of tangy lime, tender fish, and crisp vegetables offers a delightful balance of textures and flavors. Whether served as an appetizer or a main dish, ceviche is sure to impress and transport you to a seaside paradise. With minimal cooking required, this ceviche recipe is quick, easy to make, and endlessly customizable. From casual meals to special gatherings, ceviche brings the fresh taste of Latin America right to your table—ideal for summer picnics, family dinners, or any time you want a delicious, no-fuss dish.

41

Chili con Carne Recipe

Chili con carne, or simply "chili," is a beloved Tex-Mex dish known for its hearty texture, rich flavors, and a kick of spice. Translated as "chili with meat," this classic dish is traditionally made with ground beef, tomatoes, beans, and a blend of spices that give it its signature warmth and depth. While there are many variations of chili, this recipe stays true to the basics, creating a deeply flavorful and satisfying meal that's perfect for cold days, game nights, or anytime you're craving a comforting bowl of chili.

This recipe will guide you through making a traditional, slow-cooked chili con carne, with tips for customizing the spice level and adding your favorite toppings.

Ingredients

1 tbsp olive oil

1 large onion, diced

3 garlic cloves, minced

1 lb. ground beef (or ground pork or turkey)

1 large-bell pepper, diced (red or green)

1 jalapeño or serrano pepper, minced (remove seeds for less heat)

2 tbsp chili powder

1 tbsp ground cumin

1 tsp paprika

1/2 tsp dried oregano

1/2 tsp cayenne pepper (optional, for extra heat)

Salt and pepper, to taste

1 can (14.5 oz) diced tomatoes

1 can (15 oz) kidney beans, drained and rinsed

1 can (15 oz) black beans, drained and rinsed (optional)

1 cup beef broth (or more if needed)

1 tbsp tomato paste

1 tsp sugar (optional, to balance acidity)

Optional Toppings:

Shredded cheese

Sour cream or Greek yogurt

Chopped green onions

Fresh cilantro

Sliced jalapeños

Tortilla chips or cornbread on the side

Step-by-Step Instructions

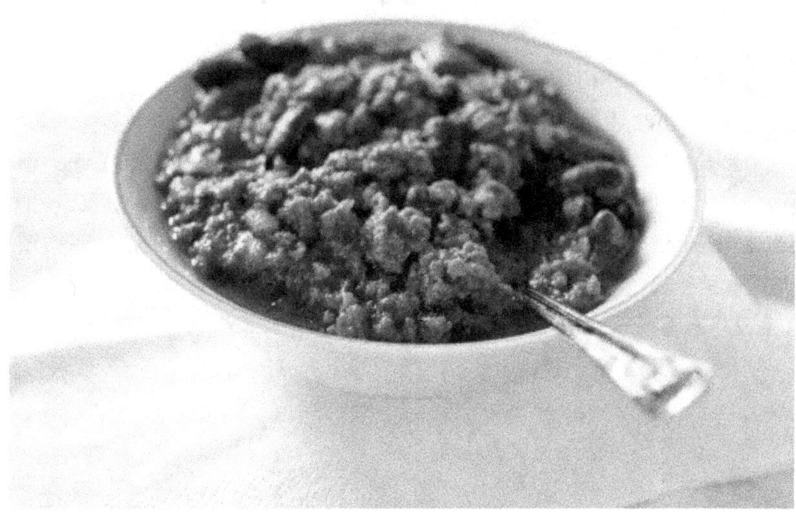

1. SAUTÉ THE AROMATICS

In a large pot or Dutch oven, heat the olive oil over medium heat. Add the diced onion and cook for about 5 minutes, or until softened and translucent. Add the minced garlic and cook for another minute, stirring frequently, until fragrant.

2. Brown the Ground Beef

Add the ground beef to the pot, breaking it up with a spoon as it cooks. Brown the meat for about 5-7 minutes, or until no longer pink. Drain any excess fat from the pot if needed.

3. Add the Vegetables and Spices

Add the diced bell pepper and minced jalapeño to the pot, stirring to combine with the beef and onions. Sprinkle in the chili powder, ground cumin, paprika, oregano, cayenne pepper (if using), salt, and pepper. Stir well to coat the meat and vegetables in the spices, cooking for about 2-3 minutes to release the flavors.

4. Add the Tomatoes, Beans, and Broth

Pour in the diced tomatoes, kidney beans, black beans (if using), beef broth, and tomato paste. Stir everything together until well combined. Add a teaspoon of sugar if you prefer slightly sweeter chili to balance the acidity of the tomatoes.

5. Simmer the Chili

Bring the chili to a boil, then reduce the heat to low. Cover the pot and let the chili simmer for at least 30 minutes, or up to 2 hours for a richer flavor, stirring occasionally. Add more beef broth if the chili becomes too thick.

6. Taste and Adjust

Before serving, taste the chili and adjust the seasoning as needed with more salt, pepper, or spices. For extra heat, you can add a dash of hot sauce or more cayenne pepper.

7. Serve and Garnish

Ladle the chili into bowls and top with your favorite garnishes, such as shredded cheese, sour cream, green onions, or fresh cilantro. Serve with tortilla chips, cornbread, or warm bread for a complete meal.

Enjoy your bowl of chili con carne while it's hot and flavorful!

Tips for Perfect Chili con Carne

Brown the Meat Well: Browning the ground beef adds depth and a slightly caramelized flavor to the chili.

Adjust the Heat: For a milder chili, omit the jalapeño and cayenne. For spicier chili, add more jalapeños or hot sauce.

Simmer for Longer Flavor: The longer the chili simmers, the more the flavors meld together. If you have time, simmer for 1-2 hours.

Balance the Acidity: If the chili tastes too acidic, a small amount of sugar can help balance the flavors.

Variations of Chili con Carne

Chili con carne is versatile, and you can customize it based on your preferences or dietary needs:

No-Bean Chili: Traditional Texas-style chili often excludes beans. Simply skip the beans and add extra beef for a meatier version.

Turkey or Chicken Chili: Substitute ground beef with ground turkey or chicken for a lighter version.

Vegetarian Chili: Use plant-based ground meat and add more beans or vegetables like zucchini, carrots, or mushrooms.

Sweet Potato Chili: Add diced sweet potatoes for extra texture and natural sweetness that complements the spices.

Serving Suggestions

Chili con carne is delicious on its own, but here are some classic sides and accompaniments:

Cornbread: A slice of cornbread is perfect for soaking up the flavors of the chili.

Tortilla Chips: Serve with crunchy tortilla chips for scooping or crumbling on top.

Rice: A side of rice makes a hearty meal and pairs well with chili.

Baked Potatoes: Top baked potatoes with a spoonful of chili for a comforting combo.

The Origins of Chili con Carne

Chili con carne has a rich history in Tex-Mex cuisine, believed to have originated in the southwestern United States, specifically in Texas. While its exact origins are debated, chili became popular in the 19th century, especially among cowboys and working-class families, who enjoyed its affordable and filling nature. Traditional Texas chili was meat-heavy, omitting beans and tomatoes, but over time, beans, tomatoes, and a variety of spices were added, giving us the beloved chili we know today.

Frequently Asked Questions

Q: Can I make chili con carne in advance?

Yes! In fact, chili often tastes better the next day as the flavors meld together. Store it in an airtight container in the refrigerator for up to 4 days and reheat it on the stove.

Q: Can I freeze chili con carne?

Absolutely. Chili freeze well for up to 3 months. Let it cool completely, then transfer to a freezer-safe container. Thaw in the refrigerator before reheating.

Q: What can I use if I don't have beef broth?

If you don't have beef broth, chicken broth, vegetable broth, or even water can be used. Adding a bit of tomato paste will still give it a rich flavor.

Q: How do I thicken chili?

If your chili is too thin, let it simmer uncovered to allow the liquid to reduce. Alternatively, you can mash some of the beans or add a bit of cornstarch slurry.

Why You'll Love This Chili con Carne Recipe

This chili con carne recipe is packed with robust flavors, thanks to the blend of spices, fresh vegetables, and slow-cooked ground beef. It's the perfect balance of smoky, spicy, and savory flavors, with a comforting texture that warms you up from the inside out. Whether you're serving it for a crowd or enjoying it as a weeknight dinner, chili con carne is versatile, filling, and endlessly customizable. Top it with your favorite garnishes, pair it with warm cornbread, and enjoy this classic dish that brings together the best of Tex-Mex comfort food.

42

Huevos Rancheros Recipe

Huevos rancheros is a traditional Mexican breakfast dish that combines fried eggs, a spicy tomato-based salsa, warm tortillas, and a variety of toppings to create a satisfying and delicious meal. The name "huevos rancheros" translates to "rancher's eggs," as it was traditionally enjoyed by farmers and ranch workers as a hearty breakfast to fuel them for the day ahead. Today, huevos rancheros is enjoyed worldwide as a flavorful and filling breakfast or brunch option.

This recipe will guide you through making authentic huevos rancheros with homemade salsa, fried eggs, and the perfect combination of toppings for a memorable breakfast experience.

Ingredients

For the Salsa:

1 tbsp olive oil

1/2 onion, diced

1-2 garlic cloves, minced

2-3 medium tomatoes, diced (or one can of diced tomatoes)

1 jalapeño or serrano pepper, minced (remove seeds for less heat)

Salt and pepper, to taste

1/2 tsp ground cumin (optional)

1/4 cup fresh cilantro, chopped

For the Huevos Rancheros:

4 large eggs

4 corn tortillas (or flour tortillas if preferred)

1/2 cup of refried beans (optional, for a heartier dish)

Salt and pepper, to taste

1 tbsp vegetable oil or butter

Optional Toppings:

Crumbled queso fresco or shredded cheese

Sliced avocado or guacamole

Fresh cilantro, chopped

Sour cream or Mexican crema

Hot sauce

Sliced green onions or diced red onion

Step-by-Step Instructions

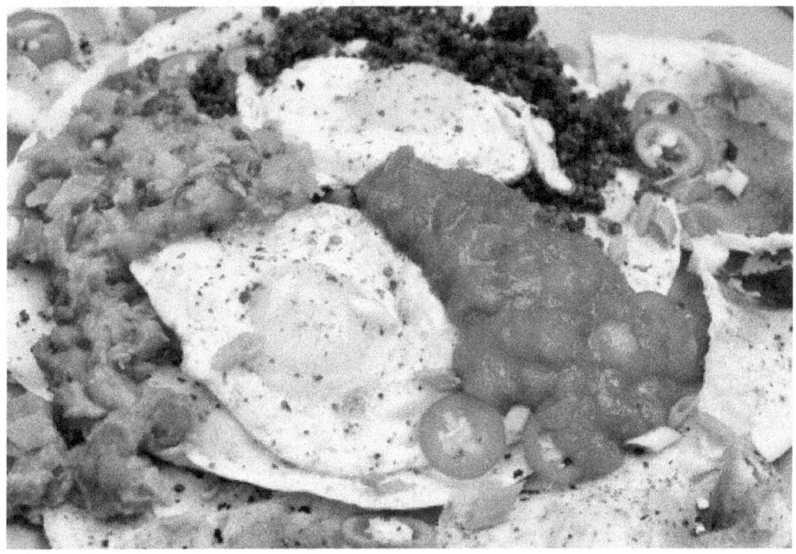

1. MAKE THE SALSA

In a skillet, heat the olive oil over medium heat. Add the diced onion and cook until softened, about 3-4 minutes. Add the minced garlic and cook for another 30 seconds, or until fragrant.

Add the diced tomatoes, minced jalapeño, salt, pepper, and cumin. Let the salsa simmer for about 5-10 minutes, until the tomatoes break down and the mixture thickens slightly. Stir in the chopped cilantro and adjust seasoning as needed. Remove from heat and set aside.

2. Prepare the Tortillas

In a separate skillet, heat a small amount of oil over medium heat. Warm each tortilla for about 1-2 minutes on each side, until soft and slightly crispy. If you like, you can keep the tortillas warm in a low oven while you prepare the eggs.

3. Fry the Eggs

In the same skillet, add a bit of vegetable oil or butter and heat over medium-low heat. Crack the eggs into the skillet, seasoning with a little salt and pepper, and cook until the whites are set but the yolks are still runny (about 3-4 minutes for sunny-side-up eggs). If you prefer firmer yolks, cook the eggs a bit longer.

4. Assemble the Huevos Rancheros

To assemble, spread a spoonful of refried beans (if using) on each tortilla, then place a warm tortilla on each plate. Top each tortilla with a fried egg, followed by a generous spoonful of the salsa.

5. Add Toppings and Serve

Finish with your choice of toppings, such as crumbled queso fresco, sliced avocado, fresh cilantro, sour cream, and a dash of hot sauce for extra heat. Serve immediately while warm, with extra salsa on the side.

Enjoy your huevos rancheros with warm tortillas, a side of rice, or fresh fruit for a complete and satisfying meal.

Tips for Perfect Huevos Rancheros

Use Fresh Ingredients: Fresh tomatoes and cilantro add a bright, authentic flavor to the salsa. If using canned tomatoes, go for a quality brand.

Adjust the Spice: For a milder dish, remove the seeds from the jalapeño or use a milder pepper like poblano. For more heat, leave the seeds in or add extra chili.

Cook the Eggs to Your Liking: Traditional huevos rancheros are served with runny yolks, but feel free to cook the eggs as you prefer.

Serve Immediately: Huevos rancheros are best enjoyed fresh, while the tortillas are warm, and the eggs are hot.

Variations of Huevos Rancheros

While classic huevos rancheros is simple and delicious on their own, here are some ways to add variety:

Huevos Divorciados: This variation uses two different sauces—one red and one green (salsa roja and salsa verde)—over each egg, making for a colorful plate.

Add Chorizo: Sauté Mexican chorizo in the skillet before adding the eggs for extra flavor and a protein boost.

Breakfast Bowl: Serve the huevos rancheros ingredients as a bowl with rice or quinoa for a heartier breakfast.

Vegetable Huevos Rancheros: Add sautéed bell peppers, zucchini, or mushrooms to the salsa for extra flavor and nutrients.

Serving Suggestions

Huevos rancheros is a filling meal on its own, but here are some side ideas to create a complete Mexican-inspired breakfast:

Mexican Rice: Serve a side of Mexican rice to round out the meal.

Fresh Fruit: Fresh fruit like mango, pineapple, or melon provides a refreshing contrast to the spicy flavors.

Refried Beans or Black Beans: A side of refried or black beans complements the flavors and adds extra protein.

Tostadas or Tortilla Chips: Offer crunchy tostadas or tortilla chips for scooping up the salsa and beans.

The Origins of Huevos Rancheros

Huevos rancheros originated in rural Mexico, where it was traditionally enjoyed by ranch workers for breakfast. The dish was made using simple, readily available ingredients, and its filling nature helped workers start their day with energy. Over time, huevos rancheros became a staple in Mexican cuisine and is now enjoyed worldwide as a classic Mexican breakfast. The combination of fried eggs, spicy salsa, and warm tortillas is not only delicious but also a reflection of Mexican culinary heritage.

Frequently Asked Questions

Q: Can I make the salsa in advance?

Yes, the salsa can be made in advance and stored in the refrigerator for up to 3 days. Reheat gently on the stove before serving.

Q: Can I use store-bought salsa?

Absolutely! While homemade salsa adds a special touch, a good-quality store-bought salsa can save time and is still delicious.

Q: Can I make huevos rancheros vegetarian?

Huevos rancheros are naturally vegetarian if made with eggs and vegetables only. Just skip the chorizo or other meat additions.

Q: Can I use flour tortillas instead of corn?

Yes, you can use flour tortillas if you prefer, though corn tortillas are traditional. Flour tortillas will add a slightly softer texture.

Why You'll Love This Huevos Rancheros Recipe

This huevos rancheros recipe brings together the classic flavors of Mexico with simple, wholesome ingredients. With its runny eggs, warm tortillas, and zesty homemade salsa, each bite is filled with comforting flavors and fresh textures. The salsa is vibrant and slightly spicy, while the toppings add layers of creaminess, freshness, and crunch. Perfect for a weekend breakfast, brunch, or even a weeknight dinner, huevos rancheros is versatile, easy to make, and endlessly satisfying. Try this recipe for a taste of authentic Mexican cuisine that's both nourishing and bursting with flavor!

43

Salsa Recipe

Mexican salsa, or salsa Mexicana, is a classic and versatile condiment that brings brightness, heat, and depth of flavor to any dish. From tacos to tortilla chips, this salsa is perfect as a dip or as a topping for a wide range of Mexican foods. Made with fresh tomatoes, onions, cilantro, lime juice, and a touch of heat from jalapeños, salsa Mexicana is quick and easy to prepare. This recipe covers how to make a fresh, authentic Mexican salsa at home.

Ingredients

4 ripe Roma tomatoes, finely diced

1/2 small onion, finely diced (white or red onion)

1-2 jalapeño or serrano peppers, finely chopped (remove seeds for less heat)

1/4 cup fresh cilantro, chopped

Juice of 1 lime (about 2 tbsp)

Salt, to taste

Optional Additions:

1 garlic clove, minced

A pinch of cumin for extra depth

1/2 tsp sugar to balance acidity (if needed)

Step-by-Step Instructions

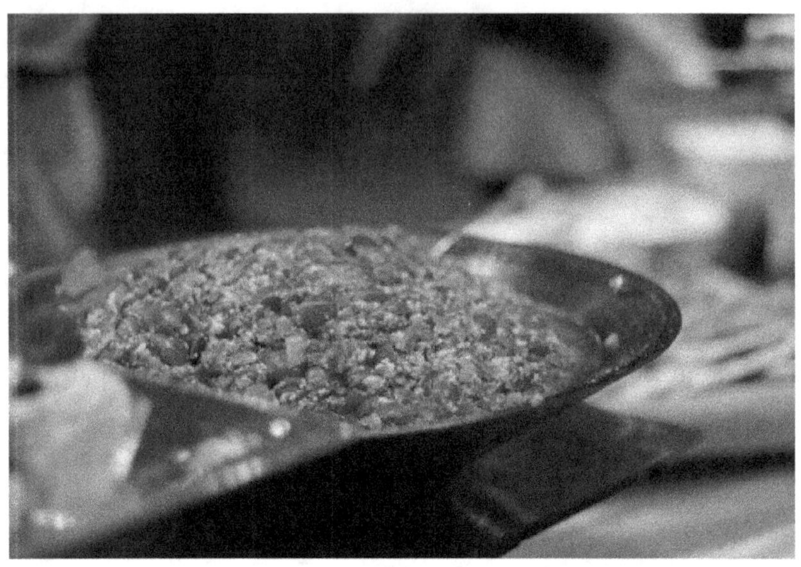

1. PREPARE THE INGREDIENTS

Dice the tomatoes, onion, and jalapeño (or serrano pepper) into small, even pieces. For a spicier salsa, leave the seeds in the jalapeño; for a milder version, remove the seeds before dicing.

2. Mix the Ingredients

In a medium bowl, combine the diced tomatoes, onion, jalapeño, and fresh cilantro. Add the lime juice and salt, stirring well to combine. Adjust the seasoning to taste, adding more lime juice, salt, or heat if desired.

3. Let the Salsa Rest (Optional)

For best results, let the salsa sit in the refrigerator for at least 10-15 minutes before serving. This allows the flavors to meld together.

4. Serve and Enjoy

Serve your fresh Mexican salsa in a bowl alongside tortilla chips, or use it as a topping for tacos, burritos, grilled meats, or any other Mexican-inspired dish.

Tips for Perfect Mexican Salsa

Use Fresh Ingredients: Fresh, ripe tomatoes and fresh lime juice make a huge difference in flavor. Roma tomatoes are ideal because they are firm and less watery.

Adjust the Spice: Jalapeños provide mild heat, while serrano peppers are spicier. You can add or reduce the number of peppers based on your spice preference.

Balance the Acidity: If the salsa tastes too acidic, add a pinch of sugar to mellow it out.

Make it Chunky or Smooth: This recipe yields a chunky salsa, but you can pulse the ingredients in a food processor for a smoother consistency if you prefer.

Variations of Mexican Salsa

While the classic version is delicious on its own, here are some fun variations to try:

Roasted Salsa: Roast the tomatoes, onions, and peppers under a broiler or on a grill until slightly charred. Then, chop and combine with the other ingredients for a smoky, rich flavor.

Pico de Gallo: A chunkier version of this salsa with less liquid, often used as a topping. To make pico de gallo, drain some of the tomato juice before mixing the ingredients.

Salsa Verde: Swap the tomatoes for tomatillos and blend with fresh cilantro, lime, and jalapeños for a bright green salsa with a slightly tangy flavor.

Fruit-Infused Salsa: Add diced mango, pineapple, or peach for a touch of sweetness that complements the spiciness.

Serving Suggestions

Mexican salsa is incredibly versatile and pairs well with many dishes. Here are some ways to serve it:

With Tortilla Chips: The classic pairing for fresh salsa, perfect for dipping.

On Tacos: Spoon salsa over tacos for a burst of fresh flavor.

With Grilled Meats: Use as a topping for grilled chicken, steak, or fish.

As a Side: Serve with enchiladas, burritos, or rice bowls to add freshness to the meal.

The Origins of Mexican Salsa

Salsa has deep roots in Mexican cuisine and dates to the Aztec, Inca, and Mayan civilizations, who made similar sauces from tomatoes, chiles, and other ingredients. Over centuries, Mexican salsa has evolved with regional varieties that reflect the local ingredients and flavors of different areas in Mexico. Today, it's a staple condiment in Mexican cuisine and is enjoyed around the world for its fresh, bold flavors and versatility.

Frequently Asked Questions

Q: Can I make salsa in advance?

Yes, salsa can be made a day in advance. Store it in an airtight container in the refrigerator for up to 3 days. The flavors actually improve as the salsa sits, making it even tastier.

Q: Can I use canned tomatoes?

While fresh tomatoes are best for salsa, you can use canned tomatoes in a pinch. Opt for diced tomatoes with no added salt or seasoning and drain them before mixing.

Q: How do I make salsa less spicy?

To reduce the spice, remove the seeds and membranes from the jalapeño, or use a mild pepper like a poblano. You can also add more tomatoes to dilute the heat.

Q: How long does homemade salsa last in the refrigerator?

Homemade salsa can be stored in the refrigerator for up to 3-4 days. If the salsa becomes watery, simply stir before serving.

Why You'll Love This Mexican Salsa Recipe

This fresh Mexican salsa recipe is vibrant, easy to make, and adaptable to your taste. With its mix of juicy tomatoes, zesty lime, and fresh herbs, each bite is bursting with flavor. Whether you're using it as a dip, topping, or side, this salsa adds a touch of brightness and spice to any meal. Perfect for gatherings, taco nights, or as a refreshing snack, this authentic Mexican salsa is sure to become a favorite in your kitchen. Enjoy it with friends, family, or simply on your own with a big bowl of tortilla chips!

44

Sopa de Tortilla Recipe

Sopa de tortilla, also known as tortilla soup, is a traditional Mexican soup with a rich tomato-based broth, crispy tortilla strips, and bold flavors. It's typically garnished with avocado, cheese, and crema for added texture and flavor. Sopa de tortilla is warm, satisfying, and surprisingly easy to make, making it a wonderful addition to any meal or a perfect standalone dish.

This recipe will guide you through making authentic sopa de tortilla with homemade fried tortilla strips and all the delicious toppings that make this soup a Mexican classic.

Ingredients

For the Soup:

1 tbsp vegetable oil

1 small onion, diced

2 garlic cloves, minced

4 ripe Roma tomatoes, diced (or one 14.5 oz can of diced tomatoes)

1-2 chipotle peppers in adobo, chopped (adjust to taste)

1 tsp ground cumin

Salt and pepper, to taste

4 cups chicken or vegetable broth

Fresh cilantro, a handful

For the Tortilla Strips:

4-6 corn tortillas, cut into thin strips

Vegetable oil, for frying

Toppings:

1 avocado, diced

1/2 cup crumbled queso fresco or shredded Monterey Jack cheese

1/4 cup Mexican crema or sour cream

Fresh cilantro leaves

Lime wedges

Step-by-Step Instructions

1. Make the Tortilla Strips

In a skillet, heat about 1/4 inch of vegetable oil over medium heat. Once the oil is hot, add the tortilla strips in small batches, frying until they are golden brown and crispy, about 1-2 minutes per batch. Remove the strips with a slotted spoon and drain them on a paper towel-lined plate. Sprinkle with a little salt and set aside.

Alternatively, for a lighter option, you can bake the tortilla strips. Spread them on a baking sheet, lightly brush with oil, and bake at 375°F (190°C) for 10-15 minutes, or until crispy and golden, turning halfway through.

2. Prepare the Soup Base

In a large pot, heat the vegetable oil over medium heat. Add the diced onion and cook until softened, about 4-5 minutes. Add the garlic and cook for another minute, until fragrant.

Stir in the diced tomatoes, chipotle peppers, and ground cumin. Cook for 5-7 minutes, stirring occasionally, until the tomatoes start to break down and the flavors meld together.

3. Blend the Soup (Optional)

For a smoother soup, transfer the tomato mixture to a blender and blend until smooth. You can also use an immersion blender directly in the pot. Blending is optional, but it creates a more uniform and creamy texture.

4. Simmer the Soup

Return the soup to the pot (if using a blender) and add the chicken or vegetable broth. Bring to a boil, then reduce the heat and let it simmer for 15-20 minutes. Season with salt and pepper to taste. Add fresh cilantro for extra flavor, letting it simmer for another 2-3 minutes before removing it from the soup.

5. Serve the Sopa de Tortilla

To serve, ladle the hot soup into bowls. Add a handful of crispy tortilla strips on top, along with diced avocado, crumbled queso fresco, a dollop of crema, and fresh cilantro. Serve with lime wedges on the side for a burst of citrusy brightness.

Enjoy your sopa de tortilla while it's warm, with all the toppings for added texture and flavor!

Tips for Perfect Sopa de Tortilla

Use Fresh Tomatoes if Possible: Fresh, ripe tomatoes give the best flavor, but canned tomatoes work well if you're short on time or out of season.

Adjust the Heat: Chipotle peppers add smoky heat. Start with one pepper and add more as desired.

Blend for a Smoother Texture: Blending the soup base creates a smoother, more consistent texture, which is traditional in many versions of sopa de tortilla.

Add Toppings Just Before Serving: To keep the tortilla strips crispy, add them to the soup right before serving.

Variations of Sopa de Tortilla

While the classic version of tortilla soup is delicious as is, here are a few ways to customize it:

Chicken Tortilla Soup: Add shredded rotisserie chicken or cooked chicken breast to make the soup heartier.

Vegetarian Tortilla Soup: Use vegetable broth and add extra vegetables, like corn, zucchini, or bell peppers, for more flavor and nutrition.

Creamy Tortilla Soup: Stir in a splash of heavy cream or coconut milk at the end for a richer, creamier version.

Tomatillo Tortilla Soup: Replace tomatoes with tomatillos for a tangy twist and a different flavor profile.

Serving Suggestions

Sopa de tortilla can be enjoyed on its own or served with other Mexican-inspired dishes for a full meal:

Mexican Rice: Serve a side of Mexican rice for a complete, comforting meal.

Tostadas or Tortilla Chips: For extra crunch, serve with tostadas or tortilla chips on the side.

Salad: A fresh salad with avocado, tomato, and lime dressing pairs well with the soup's flavors.

Grilled Corn (Elote): Add Mexican-style street corn on the cob for a flavorful side dish.

The Origins of Sopa de Tortilla

Sopa de tortilla is a traditional Mexican soup believed to have originated in the central region of Mexico, particularly in and around Mexico City. Known for its simplicity, the soup was created as a way to use up leftover tortillas by frying them and adding them to a flavorful broth. Today, sopa de tortilla is enjoyed across Mexico, often with a variety of toppings that add richness and texture to the dish.

Frequently Asked Questions

Q: Can I make sopa de tortilla in advance?

Yes, the soup base can be made in advance and stored in the refrigerator for up to 3 days. Reheat gently on the stove and add fresh tortilla strips and toppings just before serving.

Q: How can I make the soup spicier?

To increase the heat, add extra chipotle peppers, jalapeño, or even a splash of hot sauce. Adjust the spice level to your preference.

Q: Can I use flour tortillas instead of corn tortillas?

Corn tortillas are traditional and add a distinct flavor and texture. However, you can use flour tortillas if that's what you have on hand, though the taste will be slightly different.

Q: Can I freeze sopa de tortilla?

Yes, the soup base (without the toppings) can be frozen for up to 3 months. Thaw in the refrigerator overnight and reheat on the stove before adding fresh tortilla strips and toppings.

Why You'll Love This Sopa de Tortilla Recipe

This sopa de tortilla recipe is rich, flavorful, and packed with layers of comforting textures. The smoky tomato-based broth, crunchy tortilla strips, creamy avocado, and tangy lime make each spoonful a burst of vibrant Mexican flavors. It's a simple yet satisfying meal that can be customized to your taste and made as mild or spicy as you like. Perfect for cold days, cozy nights, or anytime you're in the mood for something hearty and delicious, this sopa de tortilla is an authentic Mexican dish that's easy to make and sure to become a favorite in your home.

45

Pollo Entomatado Recipe

Pollo entomatado is a traditional Mexican dish made with tender chicken simmered in a rich, flavorful tomato-based sauce. The name "entomatado" means "in tomatoes," and the sauce is the star of this dish, featuring tomatoes, garlic, onions, and aromatic spices. This comforting and delicious recipe is easy to make and perfect for family dinners or special occasions.

This recipe will guide you through making an authentic pollo entomatado with simple ingredients, creating a dish that's hearty, comforting, and bursting with Mexican flavors.

Ingredients

1 whole chicken, cut into pieces (or 6-8 chicken thighs or drumsticks)

Salt and pepper, to taste

1 tbsp vegetable oil

1 small onion, finely chopped

3 garlic cloves, minced

5 ripe Roma tomatoes, diced (or one 14.5 oz can of diced tomatoes)

1/2 cup chicken broth (or water)

1-2 jalapeño or serrano peppers, diced (optional, for heat)

1 tsp ground cumin

1/2 tsp dried oregano (preferably Mexican oregano)

Fresh cilantro, chopped (for garnish)

Lime wedges (for serving)

Step-by-Step Instructions

1. Season and Brown the Chicken

Start by seasoning the chicken pieces with salt and pepper. In a large skillet or Dutch oven, heat the vegetable oil over medium-high heat. Add the chicken pieces, skin-side down, and cook until golden brown on both sides, about 4-5 minutes per side. Remove the chicken from the skillet and set it aside.

2. Sauté the Onion and Garlic

In the same skillet, add the chopped onion and cook over medium heat until softened, about 3-4 minutes. Add the minced garlic and cook for another minute, until fragrant. Scrape up any browned bits from the bottom of the pan, as they add flavor to the sauce.

3. Make the Tomato Sauce

Add the diced tomatoes, chicken broth, jalapeño (if using), cumin, and oregano to the skillet with the onion and garlic. Stir to combine, allowing the tomatoes to break down and the sauce to come together. Let it simmer for about 5-7 minutes until the tomatoes soften and the sauce thickens slightly. If you prefer a smoother sauce, you can blend the mixture in a blender or use an immersion blender directly in the skillet.

4. Simmer the Chicken in the Sauce

Return the browned chicken pieces to the skillet, nestling them into the tomato sauce. Spoon some of the sauce over the chicken to coat it. Reduce the heat to low, cover the skillet, and let the chicken simmer in the sauce for 25-30 minutes, or until the chicken is cooked through and tender. Stir occasionally, and add a little more broth or water if the sauce becomes too thick.

5. Adjust Seasoning and Garnish

Taste the sauce and adjust the seasoning with salt and pepper as needed. Garnish with freshly chopped cilantro for a pop of color and flavor.

6. Serve and Enjoy

Serve the pollo entomatado with lime wedges on the side for an extra burst of brightness. This dish pairs wonderfully with warm corn tortillas, Mexican rice, or refried beans.

Tips for Perfect Pollo Entomatado

Use Fresh Tomatoes if Possible: Fresh, ripe tomatoes add natural sweetness and flavor. However, canned tomatoes work well if fresh tomatoes are not in season.

Brown the Chicken First: Browning the chicken before simmering adds depth and richness to the dish.

Control the Heat: For a mild dish, omit the jalapeño or serrano pepper. For a spicier version, leave the seeds in the peppers or add extra.

Simmer Slowly: Slow simmering allows the chicken to absorb the flavors of the sauce, making it tender and flavorful.

Variations of Pollo Entomatado

While this recipe is delicious as is, here are some variations to try:

Vegetable Additions: Add diced bell peppers, zucchini, or carrots to the tomato sauce for extra flavor and nutrition.

Smoky Flavor: Add a pinch of smoked paprika or use fire-roasted tomatoes for a slightly smoky flavor.

Pollo Entomatado Verde: Replace tomatoes with tomatillos for a tangy, green sauce version.

Add Potatoes: Add cubed potatoes to the sauce, allowing them to cook with the chicken for a heartier meal.

Serving Suggestions

Pollo entomatado is versatile and pairs well with a variety of Mexican-inspired sides:

Mexican Rice: A side of Mexican rice complements the flavors of the tomato sauce and adds a hearty touch.

Refried Beans or Black Beans: Serve with beans for added protein and a satisfying meal.

Corn Tortillas: Warm corn tortillas are perfect for scooping up the sauce and chicken.

Simple Green Salad: A fresh salad with lime dressing offers a nice contrast to the rich tomato sauce.

The Origins of Pollo Entomatado

Pollo entomatado has roots in traditional Mexican home cooking, where tomatoes are used in a variety of dishes. This dish showcases the use of fresh tomatoes, peppers, and aromatic spices, which are common ingredients in Mexican cuisine. Simple yet flavorful, pollo entomatado reflects the warmth and comfort of Mexican family meals and highlights the importance of tomatoes in Mexican cooking.

Frequently Asked Questions

Q: Can I make pollo entomatado in advance?

Yes, pollo entomatado can be made a day in advance. The flavors will deepen as it sits. Store it in the refrigerator and reheat it gently on the stove when ready to serve.

Q: Can I use chicken breast instead of a whole chicken?

Yes, you can use boneless chicken breasts or thighs for a quicker-cooking version. Adjust the cooking time to ensure the chicken remains tender and doesn't overcook.

Q: How do I make the sauce smoother?

If you prefer a smoother sauce, blend the tomato mixture in a blender or use an immersion blender before adding the chicken back to the skillet.

Q: Can I freeze pollo entomatado?

Yes, pollo entomatado freezes well. Store in an airtight container in the freezer for up to 3 months. Thaw in the refrigerator before reheating.

Why You'll Love This Pollo Entomatado Recipe

This pollo entomatado recipe brings together tender chicken and a rich, flavorful tomato sauce with Mexican spices. It's simple to make but full of warmth and depth, making it an ideal choice for a comforting family dinner. The tomato sauce is slightly tangy with a hint of spice, and the slow simmering ensures each piece of chicken absorbs all the delicious flavors. With its vibrant red sauce and tender chicken, pollo entomatado is a beautiful, traditional dish that's sure to satisfy. Serve it with rice, beans, or tortillas for a complete meal that's as comforting as it is delicious. Enjoy this taste of Mexican home cooking that's easy, authentic, and perfect for any occasion!

46

Shrimp in Chipotle Sauce

Shrimp in chipotle sauce, or camarones en salsa de chipotle, is a delicious Mexican dish that combines tender shrimp with a rich, smoky, and slightly spicy chipotle cream sauce. The chipotle peppers in adobo provide a deep, smoky heat that is paired perfectly with the creamy sauce and the natural sweetness of the shrimp. This dish is easy to prepare, full of flavor, and perfect for weeknight dinners or special occasions.

Here's a step-by-step recipe for authentic shrimp in chipotle sauce that brings together classic Mexican flavors in a dish that's as satisfying as it is quick to make.

Ingredients

1 lb. large shrimp, peeled and deveined

Salt and pepper, to taste

1 tbsp olive oil or vegetable oil

1/2 small onion, finely chopped

2 garlic cloves, minced

2-3 chipotle peppers in adobo sauce, finely chopped (adjust to taste)

1/2 cup heavy cream (or Mexican crema for a richer flavor)

1/4 cup milk (optional, to thin the sauce)

1 tsp tomato paste (optional, for extra depth)

Fresh cilantro, chopped (for garnish)

Lime wedges (for serving)

Step-by-Step Instructions

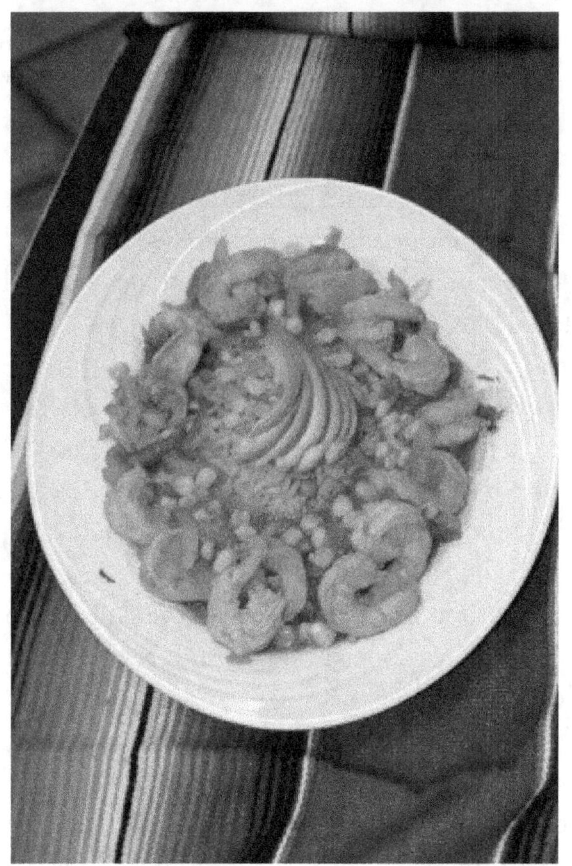

1. SEASON THE SHRIMP

Start by seasoning the shrimp with a pinch of salt and pepper. Toss gently to ensure they're evenly coated and set aside while you prepare the sauce.

2. Sauté the Onion and Garlic

In a large skillet, heat the olive oil over medium heat. Add the chopped onion and cook until softened, for about 3-4 minutes. Add the minced garlic and cook for another minute, stirring frequently, until fragrant.

3. Add the Chipotle and Cream

Stir in the chopped chipotle peppers and a little of the adobo sauce from the can. Add the heavy cream and stir well to combine. If you prefer a thinner sauce, add a splash of milk at this stage. For extra depth, you can also stir in a teaspoon of tomato paste, which will enhance the sauce's color and flavor.

4. Simmer the Sauce

Allow the sauce to simmer gently for about 5 minutes, stirring occasionally, until it thickens slightly and the flavors meld together. Taste the sauce and adjust the seasoning, adding more salt, pepper, or chipotle if desired.

5. Cook the Shrimp

Add the shrimp to the skillet, making sure they're evenly coated in the sauce. Cook for 3-4 minutes, stirring occasionally, until the shrimp turn pink and are just cooked through. Be careful not to overcook, as shrimp become rubbery when overdone.

6. Garnish and Serve

Once the shrimp are cooked, remove the skillet from the heat. Garnish with freshly chopped cilantro and serve with lime wedges on the side for added brightness.

Shrimp in chipotle sauce is best enjoyed hot, served with rice, tortillas, or a side of fresh salad.

Tips for Perfect Shrimp in Chipotle Sauce

Use Fresh Shrimp if Possible: Fresh shrimp will give the best texture and flavor. If using frozen shrimp, be sure to thaw them thoroughly before cooking.

Adjust the Spice Level: Chipotle peppers can be quite spicy, so start with one pepper and taste as you go. For a spicier sauce, add extra adobo sauce or an additional chipotle pepper.

Don't Overcook the Shrimp: Shrimp cook quickly, so keep a close eye on them to prevent them from becoming tough.

Use Mexican Crema for Authentic Flavor: Mexican crema gives the sauce a slightly tangy, rich flavor. If unavailable, heavy cream works well as a substitute.

Variations of Shrimp in Chipotle Sauce

While the classic version is delicious as is, here are some variations to try:

Shrimp and Mushroom Chipotle Sauce: Add sliced mushrooms to the sauce for extra texture and umami flavor. Sauté the mushrooms with the onions before adding the garlic.

Chipotle Cream Pasta with Shrimp: Toss the shrimp and chipotle sauce with cooked pasta for a Mexican-inspired creamy pasta dish.

Lighter Version: Use Greek yogurt or a light sour cream in place of heavy cream for a lighter, tangier version of the dish.

Add Vegetables: Bell peppers, zucchini, or spinach make great additions. Sauté them with the onion and garlic to incorporate them seamlessly into the sauce.

Serving Suggestions

Shrimp in chipotle sauce is versatile and pairs well with a variety of sides:

Mexican Rice or Cilantro-Lime Rice: A side of rice is perfect for soaking up the smoky sauce.

Warm Tortillas: Serve with warm corn or flour tortillas for scooping up the shrimp and sauce.

Fresh Salad: A side salad with avocado, tomatoes, and a light lime dressing complements the rich flavors of the chipotle sauce.

Grilled Vegetables: Grilled or roasted vegetables like zucchini, bell peppers, or asparagus add a fresh contrast.

The Origins of Chipotle Sauce

Chipotle peppers, which are smoked and dried jalapeños, are a traditional ingredient in Mexican cuisine and are especially popular in central and southern regions. The combination of chipotle peppers with cream or crema is a modern adaptation that adds a creamy richness to the smoky, spicy flavors of the peppers. This dish reflects the Mexican love for deep, layered flavors, where spicy and smoky elements are balanced by creamy, savory ingredients.

Frequently Asked Questions

Q: Can I make shrimp in chipotle sauce in advance?

Yes, you can prepare the chipotle sauce in advance and store it in the refrigerator for up to 2 days. When ready to serve, reheat the sauce in a skillet and add fresh shrimp to cook through.

Q: Can I use other seafood?

Absolutely! This recipe works well with other seafood, such as scallops, fish fillets, or even squid. Adjust the cooking time based on the seafood you use.

Q: How can I make the dish milder?

If you prefer a milder dish, use less chipotle pepper and adobo sauce, or add extra cream or milk to dilute the heat. You can also substitute the chipotle with smoked paprika for a smoky flavor without the spice.

Q: How long does leftover shrimp in chipotle sauce last?

Leftovers can be stored in the refrigerator for up to 2 days. Reheat gently on the stove over low heat to avoid overcooking the shrimp.

Why You'll Love This Shrimp in Chipotle Sauce Recipe

This shrimp in chipotle sauce recipe is a flavorful blend of smoky, spicy, and creamy elements that's both satisfying and unique. The tender shrimp in rich chipotle cream sauce creates a delightful balance of heat and creaminess, making it a standout dish that's both comforting and vibrant. Perfect for family dinners, gatherings, or date nights, this dish is quick to prepare but feels indulgent and special. Serve it with rice, tortillas, or your favorite sides, and enjoy a delicious Mexican-inspired meal that's sure to impress.

47

Flan Recipe

Flan de naranja, or orange crème caramel, is a popular dessert in Spain and Latin America that combines the classic creaminess of traditional flan with a hint of fresh orange flavor. This silky, smooth dessert is baked in a caramel-lined mold, resulting in a luscious caramel topping and a delightful citrus undertone. Flan de naranja is perfect for special occasions or as a light, elegant dessert to end any meal.

This recipe will guide you through making an authentic flan de naranja with a delicate orange flavor that pairs perfectly with the rich caramel.

Ingredients

For the Caramel:

1 cup granulated sugar

1/4 cup of water

For the Flan:

1 1/2 cups whole milk

1/2 cup heavy cream

1 cup granulated sugar

Zest of 1 large orange

1 tsp pure vanilla extract

5 large eggs

1/4 cup fresh orange juice (about half an orange)

Step-by-Step Instructions

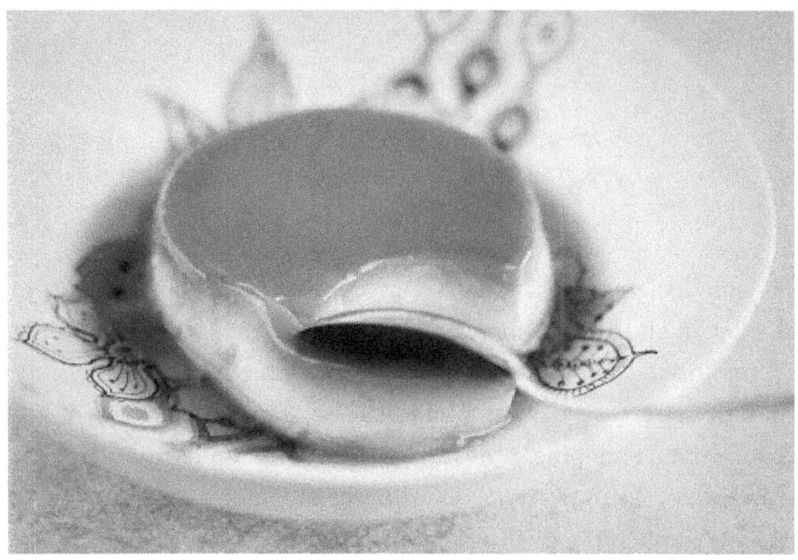

1. PREPARE THE CARAMEL

In a small saucepan over medium heat, combine the sugar and water. Stir gently to dissolve the sugar, then let the mixture cook without stirring until it turns a deep amber color, about 8-10 minutes. Swirl the pan occasionally to ensure even caramelization.

As soon as the caramel reaches the desired color, carefully pour it into a 9-inch round baking dish or flan mold, tilting the dish to evenly coat the bottom. Be careful, as the caramel will be extremely hot. Set aside to cool and harden while you prepare the flan mixture.

2. Make the Flan Mixture

In a saucepan, combine the milk, heavy cream, sugar, and orange zest. Heat over medium heat, stirring occasionally, until the sugar dissolves and the mixture is warm. Remove from heat and let it steep for a few minutes to infuse the orange flavor.

In a mixing bowl, whisk the eggs until smooth. Gradually add the warm milk mixture to the eggs, whisking constantly to avoid curdling. Stir in the vanilla extract and fresh orange juice for an extra layer of citrus flavor.

3. Strain the Mixture

For an ultra-smooth texture, pour the flan mixture through a fine-mesh strainer into a bowl. This will remove any egg solids and orange zest, resulting in a silky, creamy custard.

4. Pour and Prepare for Baking

Pour the strained mixture into the caramel-coated baking dish. Place the dish in a large roasting pan and fill the pan with hot water until it reaches halfway up the sides of the flan dish. This water bath (or bain-marie) will ensure even, gentle cooking.

5. Bake the Flan

Preheat the oven to 325°F (160°C). Carefully transfer the roasting pan to the oven and bake for 50-60 minutes, or until the flan is set but still slightly jiggly in the center. The custard will continue to firm up as it cools.

6. Cool and Refrigerate

Remove the flan from the water bath and let it cool to room temperature. Cover with plastic wrap and refrigerate for at least 4 hours, or preferably overnight, to allow the flavors to meld and the custard to fully set.

7. Unmold and Serve

To serve, run a knife around the edges of the flan to loosen it from the dish. Place a large serving plate over the flan dish and carefully invert it. Gently lift the dish to release the flan, allowing the caramel to flow over the custard.

Slice and serve the flan with a sprinkle of extra orange zest or fresh orange slices for garnish, if desired.

Tips for Perfect Flan de Naranja

Use Fresh Orange Juice: Freshly squeezed orange juice gives the flan a bright, natural flavor. Avoid bottled orange juice, as it may contain added sugars or flavors.

Don't Stir the Caramel: Once the sugar is dissolved, avoid stirring the caramel to prevent crystallization. Swirl the pan gently if needed to ensure even cooking.

Use a Water Bath: Baking the flan in a water bath prevents the custard from overcooking or curdling, resulting in a smooth texture.

Chill Thoroughly: Flan tastes best when thoroughly chilled, so make it a day ahead if possible.

Variations of Flan de Naranja

While this orange-flavored flan is delicious on its own, here are some ways to customize it:

Chocolate Flan de Naranja: Add a bit of melted dark chocolate to the custard mixture for a decadent chocolate-orange flavor.

Coconut Orange Flan: Replace half of the milk with coconut milk for a tropical twist that complements the citrus flavor.

Spiced Orange Flan: Add a pinch of cinnamon or nutmeg to the custard for a warm spice flavor.

Vanilla Bean Flan: Use a vanilla bean instead of vanilla extract for a richer, more aromatic flavor.

Serving Suggestions

Flan de naranja is elegant and versatile, and it can be served in various ways:

With Fresh Berries: Serve with fresh berries like raspberries or strawberries for a burst of color and contrast.

Whipped Cream: Add a dollop of whipped cream on top for extra richness.

Candied Orange Peel: Garnish with thin strips of candied orange peel for added citrus flavor and presentation.

Espresso or Coffee: Pair with a shot of espresso or a cup of coffee for a perfect end to a meal.

The Origins of Flan

Flan, also known as crème caramel, has a long history that dates to ancient Rome, where it was originally made with eggs and milk.

The dessert gained popularity in Spain, where it was infused with local flavors like orange and cinnamon, and it eventually spread throughout Latin America. Flan de naranja, with its bright citrus twist, is a variation that highlights the fresh flavors of oranges, which are abundant in Spanish and Latin American regions.

Frequently Asked Questions

Q: Can I make flan de naranja in individual ramekins?

Yes, you can divide the caramel and flan mixture among individual ramekins. Adjust the baking time to 30-40 minutes, checking for doneness by gently shaking the ramekins to see if the custard is set.

Q: How do I prevent bubbles in my flan?

Whisk the custard mixture gently to avoid creating bubbles. Pouring the mixture through a strainer will also help remove any bubbles and solids for a smooth texture.

Q: Can I make flan in advance?

Absolutely! Flan actually tastes better when made a day in advance, as the flavors develop, and the custard sets more firmly. Store it in the refrigerator for up to 3 days.

Q: What if my caramel hardens before I pour it into the dish?

If the caramel hardens in the pan, gently reheat it over low heat until it becomes pourable again. Be careful not to burn it.

Why You'll Love This Flan de Naranja Recipe

This flan de naranja recipe offers a luscious, creamy texture with a hint of bright orange flavor that elevates traditional flan to a new level. The smooth custard, rich caramel topping, and refreshing citrus notes create a delightful balance of flavors that's both comforting and refreshing. Whether you're preparing it for a special occasion or as a weeknight treat, this flan de naranja is sure to impress with its elegant presentation and deliciously rich taste. Make it ahead, let it chill, and enjoy a slice of this classic dessert that captures the essence of creamy, caramelized goodness with a burst of citrus.

48

Espagueti Verde Recipe

Espagueti verde, or "green spaghetti," is a popular Mexican pasta dish made with a creamy, vibrant green sauce featuring poblano peppers, cream, and fresh herbs. This dish is simple to prepare, yet it's packed with a unique, smoky flavor from the roasted poblanos. Perfect as a side dish or a main course, espagueti verde is a fantastic way to enjoy Mexican flavors in a comforting pasta dish.

Here's an authentic recipe for espagueti verde that's rich, creamy, and full of character.

Ingredients

1 lb. spaghetti

2 large poblano peppers

1 cup Mexican crema or sour cream (or heavy cream for a richer flavor)

1/2 cup milk (optional, to thin the sauce)

1/4 cup fresh cilantro, chopped

1/2 small white onion, diced

2 garlic cloves, minced

1 tbsp butter or olive oil

Salt and pepper, to taste

Queso fresco or cotija cheese, crumbled (for garnish)

Step-by-Step Instructions

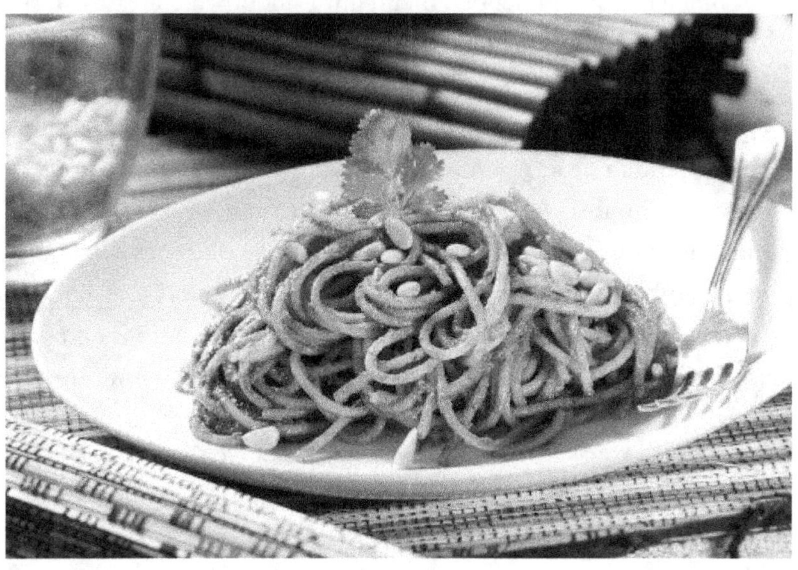

1. COOK THE SPAGHETTI

Bring a large pot of salted water to a boil. Add the spaghetti and cook according to the package instructions until al dente. Drain and set aside, reserving about 1/2 cup of the pasta cooking water.

2. Roast the Poblano Peppers

While the pasta cooks, roast the poblano peppers. Place them directly over a gas flame or on a baking sheet under the broiler, turning them occasionally, until the skins are charred and blistered on all sides, about 5-7 minutes.

Once charred, place the peppers in a plastic bag or cover them in a bowl with plastic wrap. Let them steam for about 10 minutes to make peeling easier. After steaming, peel off the charred skins, remove the stems and seeds, and chop the peppers.

3. Make the Poblano Sauce

In a blender, combine the roasted poblano peppers, Mexican crema (or sour cream), milk (if needed to thin the sauce), fresh cilantro, and a pinch of salt and pepper. Blend until smooth and creamy. Taste and adjust the seasoning as needed.

4. Sauté the Onion and Garlic

In a large skillet or saucepan, melt the butter or heat the olive oil over medium heat. Add the diced onion and cook until softened, about 3-4 minutes. Add the minced garlic and cook for another minute until fragrant.

5. Combine the Sauce and Pasta

Pour the poblano sauce into the skillet with the onions and garlic, stirring well to combine. Let the sauce simmer for 3-4 minutes to allow the flavors to meld together. If the sauce is too thick, add a bit of the reserved pasta water to reach your desired consistency.

Add the cooked spaghetti to the skillet and toss until the pasta is evenly coated in the creamy green sauce. Taste and adjust salt and pepper as needed.

6. Serve and Garnish

Transfer the espagueti verde to a serving bowl and garnish with crumbled queso fresco or cotija cheese. For extra freshness, top with a sprinkle of chopped cilantro.

Serve hot and enjoy your flavorful espagueti verde as a delicious side dish or main course!

Tips for Perfect Espagueti Verde

Roast the Poblanos Well: Properly roasting and peeling the poblano peppers is essential to achieving the smoky flavor that characterizes espagueti verde.

Adjust the Sauce Consistency: If the sauce is too thick, add a bit of milk or reserved pasta water to thin it out.

Use Mexican Crema for Authentic Flavor: Mexican crema adds a tangy richness to the sauce. If you don't have crema, sour cream or heavy cream are good substitutes.

Balance the Salt: Poblano peppers have a mild flavor, so taste the sauce and adjust the salt as needed to bring out all the flavors.

Variations of Espagueti Verde

While the classic recipe is delicious as is, here are a few variations to try:

Espagueti Verde con Pollo: Add grilled or shredded chicken for a heartier dish. Simply mix it in with the pasta and sauce for added protein.

Cheesy Espagueti Verde: Add shredded cheese, such as Monterey Jack or mozzarella, to the sauce for an extra creamy, cheesy version. Let it melt into the sauce before adding the pasta.

Spicy Espagueti Verde: For a spicy kick, add a jalapeño or serrano pepper to the sauce along with the roasted poblano peppers.

Vegetable Espagueti Verde: Add sautéed veggies like bell peppers, mushrooms, or spinach to the dish for extra texture and flavor.

Serving Suggestions

Espagueti verde is versatile and can be served in many ways:

As a Side Dish: Serve it alongside grilled meats, such as chicken, steak, or pork, for a balanced meal.

With Tostadas or Tortilla Chips: Enjoy a crunchy side with the creamy pasta.

With a Fresh Salad: A light, citrusy salad pairs well with the rich sauce.

With Sliced Avocado: Top with slices of fresh avocado for added creaminess.

The Origins of Espagueti Verde

While pasta dishes aren't traditionally Mexican, Mexican cuisine is known for blending flavors from different cultures, and espagueti verde is a perfect example of this fusion. The use of roasted poblano peppers, crema, and cilantro gives this pasta dish a distinctly Mexican flavor profile. It's a popular dish for family meals and gatherings in Mexico, where it's often enjoyed as a side dish or main course.

Frequently Asked Questions

Q: Can I make espagueti verde in advance?

Yes! You can make the sauce in advance and store it in the refrigerator for up to 2 days. Reheat the sauce gently on the stove, adding a bit of milk or water if it thickens. Then, toss it with freshly cooked pasta.

Q: Can I use other types of pasta?

Absolutely! While spaghetti is traditional, you can use any pasta shape you like, such as fettuccine, penne, or rotini.

Q: Is espagueti verde spicy?

Poblano peppers are generally mild, but if you prefer a spicier dish, you can add a jalapeño or serrano pepper to the sauce.

Q: How do I store leftovers?

Store leftovers in an airtight container in the refrigerator for up to 3 days. Reheat on the stove or in the microwave, adding a splash of milk if needed to revive the creaminess.

Why You'll Love This Espagueti Verde Recipe

This espagueti verde recipe brings together creamy, smoky, and tangy flavors that make it a unique and irresistible dish. The poblano peppers add a mild heat and distinct smokiness, while the crema and cilantro balance the flavors with richness and freshness. It's a comforting, flavorful dish that's easy to make and offers a delightful twist on traditional pasta. Whether served as a side dish, main course, or even at a potluck, espagueti verde is a standout dish that's sure to impress and satisfy. Enjoy this creamy Mexican-inspired pasta for a taste of rich, comforting flavors with a hint of spice and zest.

49

Ensalada de Nopales Recipe

Ensalada de nopales, or cactus salad, is a traditional Mexican dish made with tender nopal cactus paddles, tomatoes, onions, cilantro, and a zesty lime dressing. Nopales, or cactus paddles, are commonly used in Mexican cuisine and have a slightly tangy flavor and a crisp texture. They're packed with nutrients like fiber, vitamins, and antioxidants, making this salad both delicious and healthy. This fresh and simple dish can be enjoyed on its own, as a side, or as a topping for tacos and tostadas.

Here's how to make a classic ensalada de nopales that's refreshing, flavorful, and easy to prepare.

Ingredients

3 fresh nopales (cactus paddles), cleaned and diced

Salt, to taste

2 medium tomatoes, diced

1/4 medium white onion, finely chopped

1/4 cup fresh cilantro, chopped

1 small jalapeño or serrano pepper, minced (optional, for heat)

Juice of 2 limes

1-2 tbsp olive oil (optional, for added richness)

Freshly ground black pepper, to taste

Queso fresco or crumbled cotija cheese, for garnish (optional)

Step-by-Step Instructions

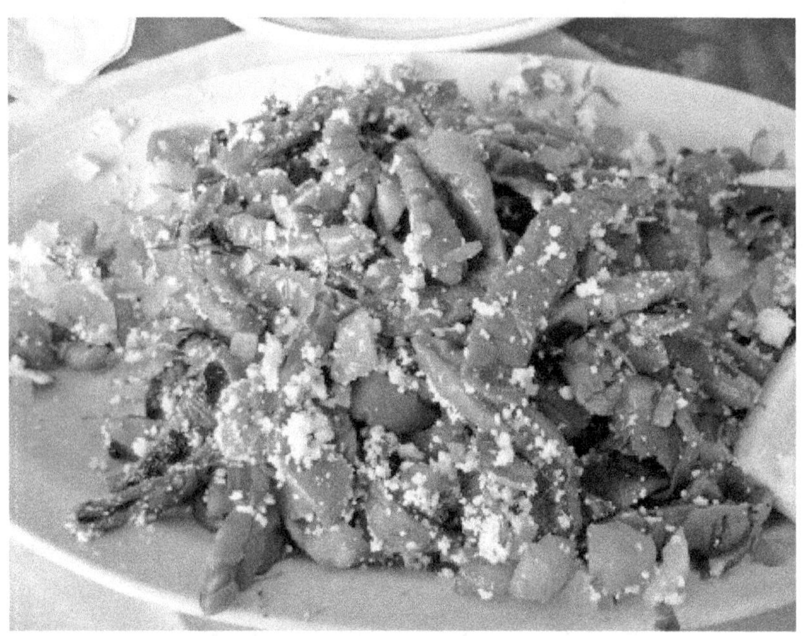

1. PREPARE THE NOPALES

To clean the nopales, use a small knife to carefully remove the thorns and spines from the cactus paddles. Rinse thoroughly under cold water.

Once cleaned, dice the nopales into small cubes. In a medium pot, bring water to a boil and add a pinch of salt. Add the diced nopales and cook for about 8-10 minutes, or until they are tender and bright green. Drain the nopales and rinse under cold water to stop the cooking process. Set aside to cool.

2. Combine the Salad Ingredients

In a large mixing bowl, combine the cooked nopales, diced tomatoes, chopped onion, cilantro, and jalapeño (if using). Stir gently to combine.

3. Make the Dressing

In a small bowl, whisk together the lime juice, olive oil (if using), salt, and freshly ground black pepper. Adjust the seasoning to taste.

4. Dress the Salad

Pour the lime dressing over the nopal mixture, tossing gently to coat everything evenly. Taste and adjust the lime, salt, or pepper if needed.

5. Garnish and Serve

Transfer the ensalada de nopales to a serving bowl and sprinkle with crumbled queso fresco or cotija cheese, if desired. Serve immediately as a fresh side dish or with tortilla chips, tostadas, or as a filling for tacos.

Tips for Perfect Ensalada de Nopales

Remove Excess Slime: Nopales release a natural, sticky substance (or "baba") when cooked. Rinsing the nopales after cooking helps reduce this. You can also add a pinch of baking soda or a few onion slices to the cooking water to reduce the slime.

Adjust the Acidity: Lime juice is a key component of the dressing. Add according to your taste.

Customize the Spice: For a milder salad, omit the jalapeño or serrano pepper. For extra heat, add a bit more or use a spicier pepper.

Use Fresh Ingredients: Fresh cilantro, juicy tomatoes, and lime juice make all the difference in flavor for this salad.

Variations of Ensalada de Nopales

While the classic version is delicious, here are some ways to change the flavors:

Add Avocado: Dice a ripe avocado and fold it into the salad for creaminess and extra nutrition.

Cucumber and Radish: Add sliced cucumbers and thinly sliced radishes for a refreshing crunch.

Ensalada de Nopales con Frijoles: Add cooked black beans or pinto beans for extra protein and a heartier salad.

Tomatillo Variation: Add diced tomatillos for a tangy, slightly sour note that complements the nopales.

Serving Suggestions

Ensalada de nopales is versatile and can be enjoyed in a variety of ways:

As a Side Dish: Serve alongside grilled meats, tacos, or enchiladas for a fresh, tangy contrast.

On Tostadas: Spread a tostada shell with refried beans and top with the ensalada de nopales for a delicious snack or light meal.

In Tacos: Add ensalada de nopales to your tacos for a refreshing twist and extra crunch.

With Tortilla Chips: Serve as a healthy dip for tortilla chips as a fun appetizer.

The Origins of Ensalada de Nopales

Nopales, or cactus paddles, have been a staple in Mexican cuisine for centuries, dating back to the time of the Aztecs. The cactus plant, also known as nopal, is native to Mexico and has become a symbol of Mexican culture and cuisine. Ensalada de nopales is a simple, fresh way to enjoy this nutritious ingredient, showcasing the traditional flavors and ingredients of Mexico. It's enjoyed widely across Mexico and has gained popularity in other parts of the world due to its health benefits and unique flavor.

Frequently Asked Questions

Q: Can I use jarred nopales?

Yes, jarred or canned nopales can be used in place of fresh nopales for convenience. Just be sure to rinse them thoroughly to remove excess salt or preservatives.

Q: How long does ensalada de nopales last?

Ensalada de nopales can be stored in an airtight container in the refrigerator for up to 2 days. The nopales may release some liquid over time, so drain before serving if needed.

Q: Is ensalada de nopales healthy?

Yes, nopales are low in calories and packed with fiber, vitamins, antioxidants, and minerals, making this salad a nutritious addition to your diet.

Q: Can I make the salad in advance?

Yes, you can prepare the salad in advance and store it in the refrigerator. However, it's best to add lime juice and cheese just before serving to keep the salad fresh.

Why You'll Love This Ensalada de Nopales Recipe

This ensalada de nopales recipe is a refreshing, healthy, and flavorful dish that celebrates the vibrant flavors of Mexican cuisine. The crisp texture of the nopales, the tangy lime dressing, and the fresh herbs make for a satisfying salad that's packed with nutrients and ideal for any occasion.

Whether you're looking for a light, nutritious side dish or a unique way to enjoy Mexican flavors, ensalada de nopales is easy to prepare, full of flavor, and a perfect addition to any meal. Enjoy this traditional Mexican salad as a refreshing and wholesome dish that's as delightful as it is nutritious!

50

Queso Fundido Recipe

Queso fundido, also known as "melted cheese," is a popular Mexican appetizer that's rich, cheesy, and irresistible. Typically made with melted cheese and flavorful toppings like chorizo, peppers, or onions, queso fundido is often served bubbling hot in a skillet with warm tortillas or tortilla chips for dipping. This dish is perfect for gatherings, game nights, or as a deliciously indulgent appetizer.

This recipe will guide you through making a classic queso fundido with chorizo and roasted peppers, bringing a burst of flavor to every gooey bite.

Ingredients

1 lb. Oaxaca cheese, Chihuahua cheese, or Monterey Jack, shredded

1/2 lb. Mexican chorizo, casing removed (or your favorite spicy sausage)

1 small white onion, finely chopped

1 poblano pepper, roasted, peeled, and diced

1 jalapeño or serrano pepper, diced (optional, for extra heat)

Fresh cilantro, chopped (for garnish)

Warm corn or flour tortillas, or tortilla chips, for serving

Step-by-Step Instructions

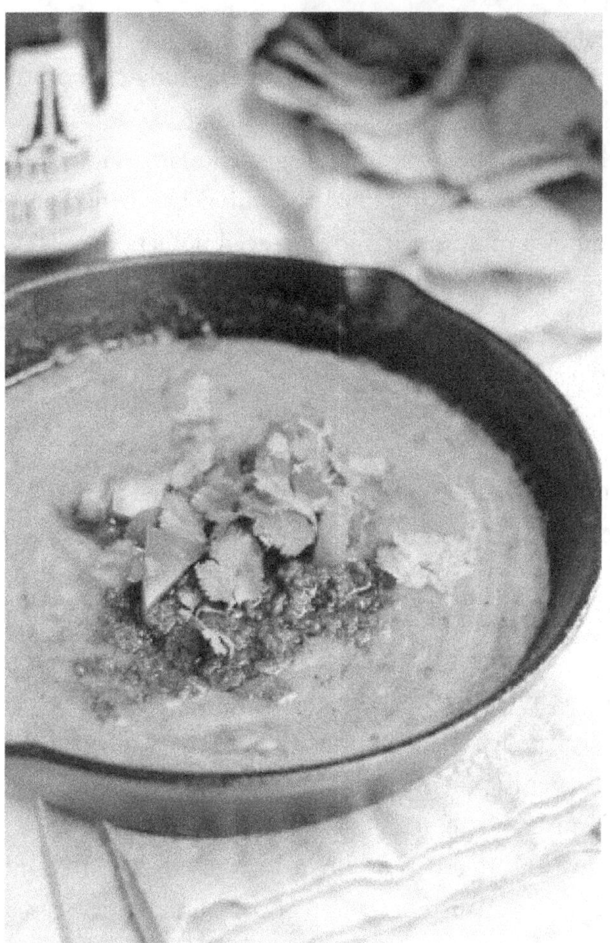

1. ROAST THE POBLANO Pepper

To prepare the poblano pepper, roast it directly over a gas flame or under the broiler until the skin is charred and blistered all over. Place the roasted pepper in a plastic bag or cover with a bowl to steam for about 10 minutes. Peel off the charred skin, remove the seeds, and dice the pepper. Set aside.

2. Cook the Chorizo and Onion

In a medium skillet over medium heat, cook the chorizo, breaking it up with a spoon, until browned and fully cooked, about 5-7 minutes. Remove any excess fat if necessary.

Add the chopped onion and jalapeño (if using) to the skillet with the chorizo, cooking until the onion is softened and translucent, about 3-4 minutes. Stir in the diced poblano pepper and cook for another 1-2 minutes to combine the flavors. Remove from heat and set aside.

3. Preheat the Oven

Preheat your oven to 400°F (200°C).

4. Assemble the Queso Fundido

In an oven-safe skillet or small baking dish, layer the shredded cheese evenly. Spoon the cooked chorizo and pepper mixture over the cheese.

5. Bake the Queso Fundido

Place the skillet or baking dish in the preheated oven and bake for 10-12 minutes, or until the cheese is fully melted and bubbling. For an extra golden top, you can switch to the broiler for the last 1-2 minutes, watching closely to prevent burning.

6. Garnish and Serve

Remove the queso fundido from the oven and sprinkle with freshly chopped cilantro for a pop of color and flavor. Serve immediately with warm tortillas or tortilla chips for dipping.

Enjoy your queso fundido while it's hot and gooey, as this is when it's at its best!

Tips for Perfect Queso Fundido

Choose the Right Cheese: For authentic queso fundido, use a melty Mexican cheese like Oaxaca or Chihuahua. If these aren't available, Monterey Jack or Mozzarella work well as substitutes.

Serve Immediately: Queso fundido is best served straight out of the oven, as the cheese can start to harden as it cools. Enjoy it while it's hot and stretchy.

Customize the Spice: For more heat, add diced jalapeño, serrano peppers, or a sprinkle of chili flakes.

Use an Oven-Safe Skillet: An oven-safe skillet, like cast iron, works well for baking and serving queso fundido.

Variations of Queso Fundido

While chorizo and peppers are classic toppings, there are many ways to customize queso fundido to suit your tastes:

Vegetarian Queso Fundido: Skip the chorizo and add sautéed mushrooms, bell peppers, or spinach for a veggie-packed version.

Queso Fundido with Shrimp: Sauté small shrimp in butter and garlic, then add them to the melted cheese for a seafood twist.

Queso Fundido con Rajas: Add strips of roasted poblano peppers (known as rajas) and caramelized onions for a smoky, mildly spicy flavor.

Four-Cheese Queso Fundido: Combine Oaxaca, Monterey Jack, queso fresco, and a touch of cheddar for a multi-cheese experience.

Serving Suggestions

Queso fundido is rich and satisfying on its own, but here are some ways to make it part of a larger meal:

With Tortillas: Serve with warm corn or flour tortillas to make mini tacos or wraps.

As a Dip: Pair with crunchy tortilla chips, or even pita chips, for dipping.

With Fresh Salsa: A spoonful of salsa or pico de gallo on top adds freshness and acidity that balances the richness.

Side Dishes: Serve alongside guacamole, fresh salsa, or Mexican rice for a complete appetizer spread.

The Origins of Queso Fundido

Queso fundido is a beloved Mexican appetizer with roots in northern Mexico. It's thought to have originated to use up bits of cheese and sausage, creating a simple yet satisfying dish that's both flavorful and comforting. Queso fundido is typically served as an appetizer or shared dish, and its popularity has spread beyond Mexico, with different regions adding their own spins and toppings.

Frequently Asked Questions

Q: Can I make queso fundido on the stovetop?

Yes! You can melt the cheese on the stovetop over low heat, stirring until smooth. Add the chorizo and peppers once the cheese is melted, then transfer to a serving dish or eat directly from the skillet.

Q: Can I reheat queso fundido?

Queso fundido is best enjoyed fresh, but you can reheat it gently in the oven or on the stovetop. Add a splash of milk if it has hardened and stir to bring back the creamy texture.

Q: Is queso fundido the same as queso dip?

Not quite. Queso fundido is usually made with real, shredded cheese (without added cream or milk), giving it a thicker, stretchier consistency than queso dip, which often includes cream or processed cheese.

Q: How long does queso fundido stay melty?

Queso fundido will stay melty and gooey for about 10-15 minutes after it comes out of the oven, so it's best to enjoy it right away.

Why You'll Love This Queso Fundido Recipe

This queso fundido recipe combines melted, gooey cheese with the smoky, spicy flavor of chorizo and roasted poblano peppers, creating a rich and indulgent dish that's impossible to resist. With its stretchy texture and bold flavors, queso fundido is perfect for gatherings, family dinners, or as a special treat to share. Serve it with warm tortillas, chips, and your favorite toppings for a crowd-pleasing appetizer that's easy to make and even easier to enjoy. This queso fundido is more than just melted cheese—it's a taste of Mexican tradition and comfort in every bite.

51

Rollo de Fresa Recipe

Rollo de fresa, or strawberry roll cake, is a delightful dessert that combines a soft, fluffy sponge cake with a creamy filling and fresh strawberries. This light and elegant dessert is perfect for spring and summer, when strawberries are in season. The cake is rolled up with the filling inside, creating beautiful swirls of cake and strawberries in each slice. Rollo de fresa is a treat that's sure to impress, yet it's surprisingly easy to make at home.

Here's an easy-to-follow recipe for an authentic rollo de fresa that's sweet, light, and packed with strawberry flavor.

Ingredients

For the Cake:

4 large eggs, at room temperature

1/2 cup granulated sugar

1 tsp vanilla extract

1/4 cup of milk, at room temperature

1/2 cup all-purpose flour, sifted

1/2 tsp baking powder

A pinch of salt

For the Filling:

1 cup heavy whipping cream, cold

2 tbsp powdered sugar

1 tsp vanilla extract

1 cup fresh strawberries, diced

For Garnish:

Powdered sugar, for dusting

Fresh strawberries, for decorating
Step-by-Step Instructions

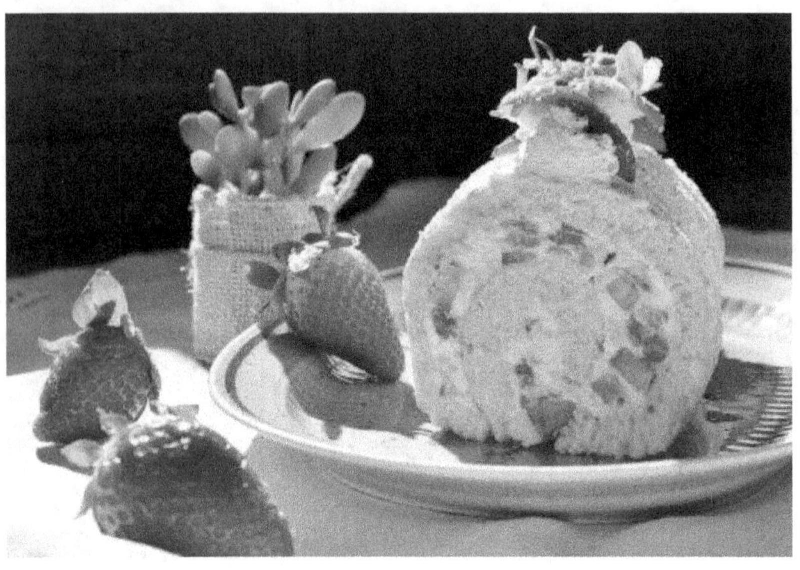

1. PREHEAT THE OVEN and Prepare the Pan

Preheat your oven to 350°F (175°C). Line a 10x15-inch baking pan or jelly roll pan with parchment paper, and lightly grease it to prevent sticking.

2. Make the Sponge Cake

In a large mixing bowl, beat the eggs with an electric mixer on high speed until they are thick, pale, and doubled in volume, about 5-6 minutes. Gradually add the sugar, continue to beat until the mixture is light and fluffy. Add the vanilla extract and milk and mix until just combined.

In a separate bowl, sift together the flour, baking powder, and salt. Gently fold the dry ingredients into the egg mixture with a spatula, being careful not to deflate the batter.

3. Bake the Cake

Pour the batter into the prepared pan, spreading it evenly with a spatula. Bake for 10-12 minutes, or until the cake is light golden and springs back when touched. Be careful not to overbake, as this can make the cake difficult to roll.

4. Roll the Cake

While the cake is still warm, place a clean kitchen towel on your work surface and dust it with powdered sugar. Carefully invert the cake onto the towel and peel off the parchment paper. Starting from one of the short ends, gently roll the cake with the towel inside. This "pre-roll" will help the cake hold its shape without cracking when it's filled. Allow the rolled cake to cool completely.

5. Prepare the Cream Filling

In a mixing bowl, beat the cold heavy whipping cream with an electric mixer until soft peaks form. Add the powdered sugar and vanilla extract and continue to beat until the cream holds stiff peaks. Be careful not to overbeat, as this can cause the cream to become grainy. Gently fold in the diced strawberries.

6. Fill and Roll the Cake

Once the cake has cooled, carefully unroll it. Spread the whipped cream and strawberry mixture evenly over the surface of the cake, leaving a small border around the edges to prevent the filling from spilling out. Carefully roll the cake back up without the towel, rolling tightly but gently to keep the filling inside.

7. Dust and Garnish

Place the rollo de fresa seam-side down on a serving plate. Dust the top with powdered sugar and garnish with additional fresh strawberries if desired.

8. Chill and Serve

Refrigerate the cake for at least 30 minutes to allow it to set. When ready to serve, slice the roll into 1-inch pieces to reveal the beautiful strawberry swirl inside. Enjoy your rollo de fresa!

Tips for Perfect Rollo de Fresa

Roll the Cake While Warm: Rolling the cake while it's still warm helps prevent cracks and makes it easier to roll later with the filling.

Use Fresh Strawberries: Fresh, ripe strawberries provide the best flavor and texture. Frozen strawberries can release too much moisture, making the filling runny.

Chill Before Slicing: Refrigerating the cake for at least 30 minutes before slicing helps it hold its shape and makes cleaner cuts.

Dust with Powdered Sugar Last: Wait until just before serving to dust with powdered sugar, as it can absorb moisture from the cake and disappear if added too early.

Variations of Rollo de Fresa

While classic rollo de fresa is delicious as is, here are some fun ways to customize it:

Chocolate Rollo de Fresa: Add 2 tbsp of cocoa powder to the cake batter for a chocolate-flavored cake, pairing perfectly with the strawberry filling.

Lemon Strawberry Roll: Add a teaspoon of lemon zest to the cake batter and a bit of lemon juice to the whipped cream for a bright, citrusy flavor.

Strawberry Cream Cheese Filling: Use a mix of cream cheese and whipped cream for a richer, tangy filling that pair well with strawberries.

Berry Mix Roll: Add other fresh berries like raspberries or blueberries to the filling for a mixed berry twist.

Serving Suggestions

Rollo de fresa is light and refreshing, making it a wonderful dessert for warm days or special occasions. Here are some ways to serve it:

With Extra Whipped Cream: Serve slices with a dollop of whipped cream on the side for added richness.

Chocolate Drizzle: Drizzle melted chocolate or chocolate ganache over the cake for an indulgent touch.

With Fresh Fruit: Garnish with extra fresh strawberries, blueberries, or raspberries for added color and flavor.

With Ice Cream: Serve a slice with a scoop of vanilla or strawberry ice cream for a complete dessert.

The Origins of Rollo de Fresa

While rollo de fresa may not be a traditional Mexican dessert, it has become popular in Mexican bakeries and homes, especially during the spring and summer when strawberries are abundant. This light, fruity cake is like the European Swiss roll but with a Latin twist, featuring fresh ingredients and flavors that make it a favorite for family gatherings and celebrations.

Frequently Asked Questions

Q: Can I make rollo de fresa in advance?

Yes, rollo de fresa can be made a day in advance. Store it in the refrigerator, wrapped in plastic wrap, to keep it fresh. Dust with powdered sugar just before serving.

Q: Can I use frozen strawberries?

It's best to use fresh strawberries, as frozen strawberries can release extra moisture and make the filling watery. If you must use frozen, thaw them and drain excess liquid before adding to the filling.

Q: How long does rollo de fresa last?

Rollo de fresa can be stored in the refrigerator for up to 3 days. Keep it covered to prevent it from drying out.

Q: Can I freeze rollo de fresa?

Yes, rollo de fresa can be frozen. Wrap it tightly in plastic wrap and store it in the freezer for up to 1 month. Thaw in the refrigerator overnight before serving.

Why You'll Love This Rollo de Fresa Recipe

This rollo de fresa recipe combines the airy, tender texture of sponge cake with the sweet and tangy flavor of fresh strawberries and cream. It's a light, elegant dessert that's perfect for gatherings or simply as a sweet treat for yourself. The bright strawberry flavor pairs beautifully with the soft, fluffy cake, making each slice a delightful balance of flavor and texture. Easy to make and a joy to share, rollo de fresa is a dessert that brings a little bit of sunshine to the table. Whether for a celebration or a casual get-together, this strawberry roll cake is sure to impress and satisfy.

52

Conchas Recipe

Conchas are one of the most beloved types of pan dulce (Mexican sweet bread) and a staple in Mexican bakeries. They are known for their soft, fluffy texture and distinctive shell-like topping, which is where they get their name ("concha" means "shell" in Spanish). The topping, made with sugar, butter, and flour, is often flavored with vanilla or chocolate and creates a lightly crunchy, sweet crust on the soft, pillowy bread underneath. Perfect for breakfast, a snack, or dessert, conchas are a delightful treat with coffee or hot chocolate.

Here's a classic recipe for conchas that's easy to follow and produces delicious, authentic results.

Ingredients

For the Dough:

3 1/2 cups of all-purpose flour, plus extra for kneading

1/2 cup granulated sugar

1 tsp of salt

2 1/4 tsp active dry yeast (1 packet)

1/2 cup warm milk (110°F/43°C)

3 large eggs, at room temperature

1/2 cup unsalted butter, softened and cut into pieces

For the Topping:

1/2 cup unsalted butter, softened

1/2 cup powdered sugar

1 cup all-purpose flour

1 tsp vanilla extract

1 tbsp cocoa powder (optional, for chocolate topping)

Step-by-Step Instructions

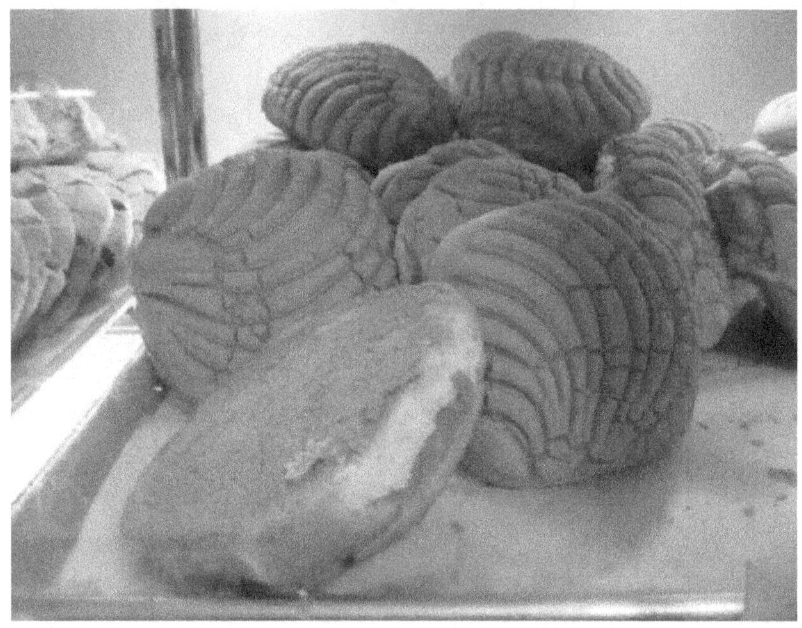

1. ACTIVATE THE YEAST

In a small bowl, combine the warm milk and yeast. Let it sit for about 5 minutes until the yeast becomes foamy. This step ensures that the yeast is active and will help the dough rise.

2. Make the Dough

In the bowl of a stand mixer fitted with the dough hook attachment, combine the flour, sugar, and salt. Add the yeast mixture and eggs and mix on low speed until the ingredients come together.

Add the softened butter, a few pieces at a time, and continue mixing until the dough is smooth and elastic, for about 10-12 minutes. The dough should be soft and slightly sticky but pull away from the sides of the bowl. If it's too sticky, add a bit more flour, 1 tablespoon at a time, until it reaches the right consistency.

3. Let the Dough Rise

Transfer the dough to a lightly greased bowl and cover it with a clean kitchen towel. Place it in a warm, draft-free spot and let it rise for 1-2 hours, or until double in size.

4. Prepare the Topping

While the dough rises, make the topping. In a medium bowl, beat the softened butter and powdered sugar together until smooth. Gradually add the flour and vanilla extract, mixing until a soft dough forms.

Divide the topping dough in half. Leave one half plain (for vanilla topping) and add cocoa powder to the other half (for chocolate topping), kneading it until the color is even.

Roll each portion of the topping dough into small balls, about 1 inch in diameter. Cover with plastic wrap and set aside.

5. Shape the Conchas

Once the dough has doubled in size, punch it down to release any air bubbles. Divide the dough into 12 equal portions and shape each portion into a smooth ball. Place the dough balls onto a baking sheet lined with parchment paper, spacing them at least 2 inches apart.

Flatten each topping ball into a disk and place it on top of each dough ball, gently pressing it down so it adheres to the dough.

6. Create the Shell Pattern

Using a small knife or a concha cutter, gently score the topping in a shell-like pattern (or any desired pattern). This step gives the conchas their traditional, shell-like appearance. Cover the conchas loosely with a towel and let them rise again for about 30-45 minutes, or until slightly puffy.

7. Bake the Conchas

Preheat your oven to 350°F (175°C). Once the conchas has risen, bake them for 18-20 minutes, or until the tops are lightly golden and the bread is cooked through. The topping should be slightly firm to the touch.

Allow the conchas to cool on a wire rack before serving.

Tips for Perfect Conchas

Use Softened Butter: For both the dough and the topping, softened butter ensures the ingredients incorporate smoothly and produce a soft texture.

Don't Overwork the Topping: Handle the topping dough gently to avoid toughening it, as you want a light, crumbly crust on top.

Let the Dough Rise Fully: Allowing the dough to rise properly results in a fluffy, airy bread that contrasts beautifully with the sweet topping.

Use a Concha Cutter for a Traditional Pattern: If you want an authentic shell pattern, concha cutters are available online and in Latin markets. Otherwise, use a small knife to create your own designs.

Variations of Conchas

Traditional conchas are delicious as is, but here are some ways to change up the flavors and textures:

Cinnamon Conchas: Add a teaspoon of ground cinnamon to the dough for a warm, spiced flavor.

Flavored Toppings: Experiment with other flavors in the topping, like almond or strawberry extract.

Fillings: Add a filling, such as dulce de leche or chocolate ganache, by creating a small indentation in the dough ball and adding a spoonful before sealing it.

Colorful Conchas: Use food coloring in the topping dough to create brightly colored conchas, a popular trend in Mexican bakeries.

Serving Suggestions

Conchas are wonderful with coffee, hot chocolate, or Mexican café de olla. Here are some additional serving ideas:

Concha Sandwich: Slice the concha in half and fill with sweet fillings like Nutella, peanut butter, or whipped cream for an extra indulgent treat.

Concha French Toast: Dip halved conchas in egg and milk mixture and cook as French toast for a unique breakfast.

Ice Cream Concha Sandwich: Slice a concha in half and fill it with ice cream for a fun and delicious dessert.

The Origins of Conchas

Conchas are part of the vast tradition of pan dulce in Mexico, which was influenced by Spanish baking techniques during colonial times. Mexican bakers combined local ingredients with European baking methods, creating a unique style of sweet bread with inventive shapes and designs. Conchas are among the most popular of these breads, enjoyed by people of all ages. They're often part of a traditional breakfast or merienda (afternoon snack) and are an enduring symbol of Mexican bakery culture.

Frequently Asked Questions

Q: Can I make conchas without a stand mixer?

Yes, you can knead the dough by hand. It will take a bit longer, around 15-20 minutes, to achieve a smooth, elastic consistency.

Q: How do I store conchas?

Store conchas in an airtight container at room temperature for up to 3 days. You can also freeze them for up to 2 months and reheat them in the oven.

Q: Can I make conchas with whole wheat flour?

Yes, you can substitute some of the all-purpose flour with whole wheat flour, though this may result in denser bread. Use 50% whole wheat flour for the best texture.

Q: Can I make the dough in advance?

Yes, you can refrigerate the dough after the first rise for up to 12 hours. Allow it to come to room temperature before shaping and baking.

Why You'll Love This Conchas Recipe

This conchas recipe delivers soft, fluffy bread with a perfectly sweet, crumbly topping. The contrasting textures and flavors make each bite a delight, and the traditional shell pattern adds a touch of artistry to the presentation. Conchas is ideal for breakfast, as a snack, or as a comforting treat to enjoy with family and friends. Making conchas from scratch is a rewarding way to experience the warmth and tradition of Mexican bakery culture at home. With this recipe, you'll enjoy an authentic taste of Mexico's beloved pan dulce, made fresh and full of love.

53

Bolillos Recipe

Bolillos are Mexico's answer to the French baguette—a small, crusty bread roll with a soft, fluffy interior. Known for their distinctive oval shape and a slight split down the middle, bolillos are versatile and enjoyed throughout Mexico as a staple bread. They're perfect for making tortas (Mexican sandwiches), dipping into soups, or enjoying with butter or jam. With a crispy crust and tender crumb, bolillos are an essential part of Mexican cuisine and are easy to make at home.

This recipe will guide you through making authentic bolillos, creating a homemade bread that's fresh, crusty, and delicious.

Ingredients

4 cups of all-purpose flour, plus extra for kneading

2 1/4 tsp active dry yeast (1 packet)

1 1/2 tsp salt

1 tbsp sugar

1 1/2 cups warm water (110°F/43°C), plus extra for brushing

2 tbsp vegetable oil

Step-by-Step Instructions

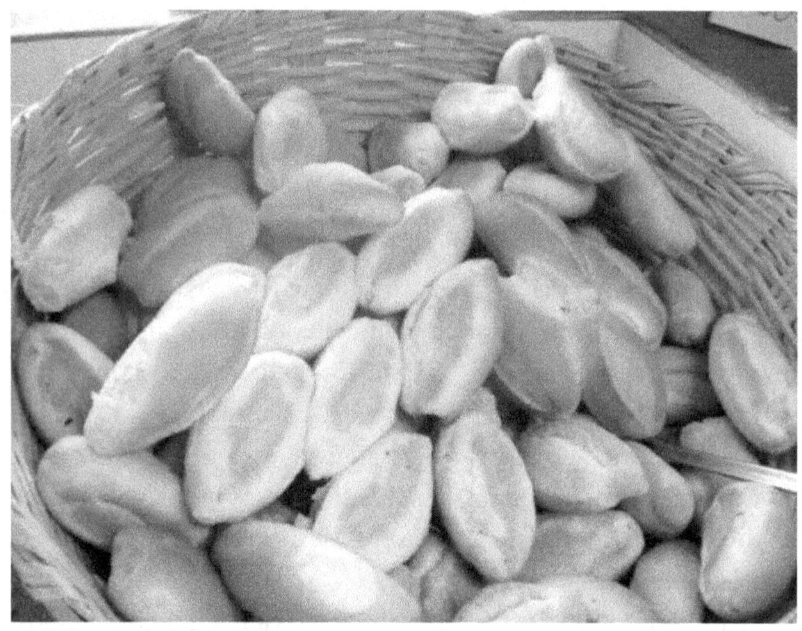

1. ACTIVATE THE YEAST

In a small bowl, combine the warm water, sugar, and active dry yeast. Let it sit for 5-10 minutes until the yeast becomes foamy. This step ensures the yeast is active and will help the dough rise.

2. Make the Dough

In a large mixing bowl or the bowl of a stand mixer fitted with the dough hook, combine the flour and salt. Add the yeast mixture and vegetable oil to the flour, and mix on low speed until the dough begins to come together.

Increase the speed to medium and continue mixing for 8-10 minutes, or until the dough is smooth, elastic, and slightly sticky. If kneading by hand, knead for about 10 minutes until the dough is stretchy and smooth. If the dough is too sticky, add a little more flour, one tablespoon at a time, until it reaches the right consistency.

3. First Rise

Place the dough in a lightly greased bowl, cover it with a clean kitchen towel, and let it rise in a warm, draft-free spot for 1-1.5 hours, or until doubled in size.

4. Shape the Bolillos

After the dough has risen, punch it down to release any air bubbles. Turn it out onto a lightly floured surface and divide it into 8 equal pieces.

To shape each bolillo, take a piece of dough and flatten it slightly. Fold the edges toward the center, pinching them to form a tight seam. Roll the dough back and forth gently to form an oval, tapering the ends slightly. Place each shaped bolillo on a baking sheet lined with parchment paper or a silicone mat, seam-side down.

5. Second Rise

Cover the shaped bolillos with a towel and let them rise for 30-45 minutes, or until they puff up slightly.

6. Preheat the Oven

Preheat your oven to 425°F (220°C). Place a baking pan filled with water on the bottom rack of the oven to create steam, which helps develop a crispy crust on the bolillos.

7. Score and Brush the Bolillos

Once the bolillos have risen, use a sharp knife or bread lame to make a shallow slash lengthwise down the center of each roll. Brush the tops lightly with water to enhance the crustiness.

8. Bake the Bolillos

Bake the bolillos in the preheated oven for 18-20 minutes, or until they are golden brown and sound hollow when tapped on the bottom. The steam from the water pan will help create a crispy, crackly crust.

9. Cool and Serve

Transfer the bolillos to a wire rack to cool before slicing or serving. Enjoy them warm with butter, or use them for sandwiches, alongside soups, or with any meal!

Tips for Perfect Bolillos

Create Steam in the Oven: Placing a pan of water in the oven while baking creates steam, which is essential for achieving a crispy crust. You can also spritz the oven with water right after placing the bolillos inside for extra steam.

Use Warm Water for Yeast: Make sure the water is warm, but not hot, to properly activate the yeast.

Shape with Tapered Ends: The traditional shape of bolillos is an oval with slightly tapered ends, so gently shape each roll to resemble this form.

Allow Proper Rising Time: Giving the dough enough time to rise in both the first and second rise ensures the rolls are light, airy, and fluffy on the inside.

Variations of Bolillos

While classic bolillos are delicious as they are, here are some variations you can try:

Whole Wheat Bolillos: Replace half of the all-purpose flour with whole wheat flour for a heartier, slightly nutty flavor.

Jalapeño-Cheddar Bolillos: Mix chopped jalapeños and shredded cheddar cheese into the dough for a spicy, savory twist.

Herbed Bolillos: Add fresh or dried herbs, such as rosemary or thyme, to the dough for an aromatic flavor.

Mini Bolillos: Make smaller bolillos by dividing the dough into 12-16 pieces instead of 8 for mini rolls that are perfect for sliders or small sandwiches.

Serving Suggestions

Bolillos are incredibly versatile and pair well with many dishes. Here are some popular ways to enjoy them:

Tortas: Bolillos are perfect for Mexican tortas. Slice them in half, fill with meats, cheese, avocado, and pickled jalapeños, and press lightly for a delicious sandwich.

Alongside Soup: Serve bolillos with Mexican soups like pozole, menudo, or caldo de pollo for a satisfying meal.

With Butter and Jam: Enjoy bolillos warm with butter, jam, or honey as a simple breakfast or snack.

For Dipping: Use bolillos to dip into salsa, guacamole, or even melted cheese for a tasty appetizer.

The Origins of Bolillos

Bolillos have their origins in France, with the baguette influencing their development in Mexico. The French introduced bread-making techniques to Mexico in the 19th century, and local bakers adapted the French baguette to create a smaller, crustier roll that has since become an iconic part of Mexican cuisine. Bolillos are often associated with the Mexican meal tradition, enjoyed at any time of day and with a variety of fillings or sides. Today, bolillos can be found in bakeries across Mexico, where they are enjoyed as an everyday staple.

Frequently Asked Questions

Q: Can I make bolillos without a stand mixer?

Yes! You can knead the dough by hand. It will take about 10-12 minutes to reach the right smooth, elastic consistency.

Q: How do I store bolillos?

Bolillos are best eaten fresh, but you can store them in an airtight container at room temperature for up to 2 days. To re-crisp the crust, heat them in a 350°F (175°C) oven for about 5 minutes.

Q: Can I freeze bolillos?

Yes, bolillos freeze well. Once cooled, wrap them tightly in plastic wrap and place them in a freezer bag. Thaw at room temperature and warm in the oven before serving.

Q: Can I use bread flour instead of all-purpose flour?

Yes, bread flour can be used and will create a slightly chewier texture. You may need to add a bit more water to the dough if using bread flour.

Why You'll Love This Bolillos Recipe

This bolillos recipe produces delicious, crusty rolls with a soft, airy interior that's perfect for sandwiches or as a side to any meal. The authentic flavor and texture make these rolls a satisfying addition to your bread-baking repertoire. Simple ingredients come together to create a homemade version of one of Mexico's most popular breads, and the crispy crust with the soft crumb makes bolillos a comforting and versatile choice. Whether you're serving them with soup, making tortas, or enjoying them with butter and jam, bolillos bring the taste of traditional Mexican bakeries to your kitchen. Freshly baked and warm, these bolillos are sure to become a favorite!

54

Tepache Recipe

Tepache is a popular Mexican drink made from fermented pineapple peels, sugar, and spices. Slightly effervescent and mildly alcoholic, tepache has a tangy, sweet flavor with hints of cinnamon and cloves. Traditionally, it's served chilled and enjoyed as a refreshing drink, especially on hot days. With a simple fermentation process, tepache is easy to make at home and a great way to use leftover pineapple peels.

Here's a traditional recipe for tepache that will give you a delicious, homemade taste of this beloved Mexican drink.

Ingredients

1 ripe pineapple (only the peel and core, but keep the flesh for another use)

8 cups of water

1 1/2 cups piloncillo (or dark brown sugar as a substitute)

1 cinnamon stick

2-3 whole cloves (optional)

Step-by-Step Instructions

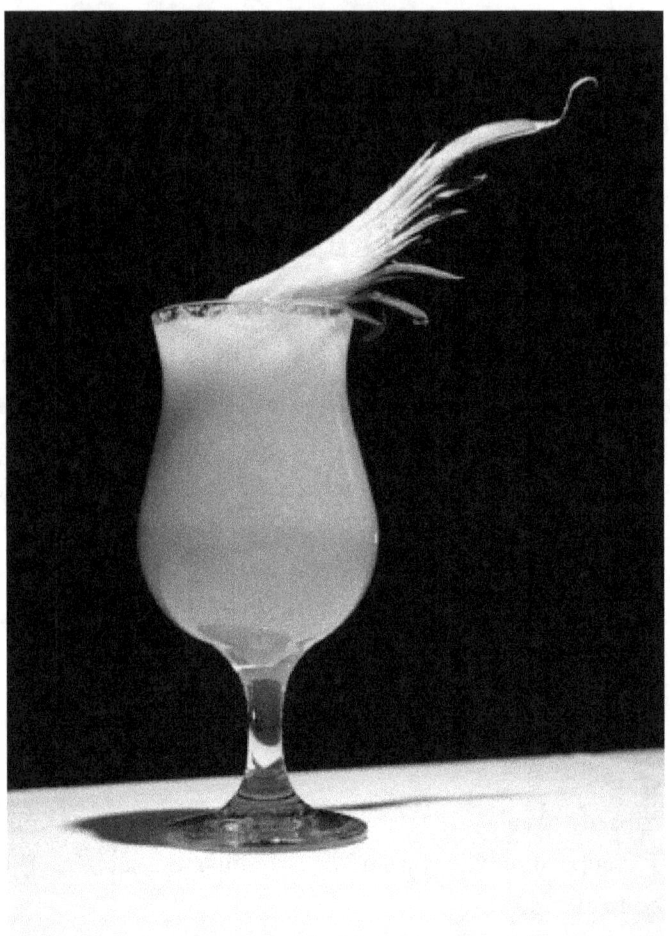

1. PREPARE THE PINEAPPLE

Start by thoroughly washing the pineapple to remove any dirt. Cut off the crown and base, then peel the pineapple. Save the flesh for another recipe or snack, as you'll only need the peel and core for this tepache recipe. Cut the peel and core into chunks.

2. Dissolve the Sugar

In a large pot, add the water and bring it to a boil. Add the piloncillo or brown sugar and stir until it completely dissolves. Remove from heat and let the sweetened water cool to room temperature.

3. Assemble the Tepache Ingredients

Place the pineapple peels and core in a large glass jar or pitcher (about 1-gallon capacity). Add the cinnamon stick and cloves, then pour the cooled sugar water over the pineapple and spices.

4. Cover and Ferment

Cover the jar loosely with a clean cloth or cheesecloth. This allows air to flow in and out, promoting natural fermentation while keeping out dust and insects. Let the mixture sit at room temperature in a cool, dark place for 2-3 days. During this time, the pineapple peels will release natural sugars, and the mixture will begin to ferment.

5. Check for Fermentation

After 2 days, taste the tepache. It should have a mildly tangy, sweet flavor with a slight effervescence. If you prefer a stronger flavor, you can let it ferment for another day, but be careful not to leave it too long, as tepache can quickly turn too sour.

6. Strain and Serve

Once the tepache has reached your desired taste, strain it through a fine-mesh sieve or cheesecloth into a clean pitcher, discarding the pineapple peels and spices. Transfer the tepache to the refrigerator to chill before serving.

7. Enjoy Your Tepache

Serve the tepache over ice for a refreshing drink. If you prefer extra fizz, you can let the strained tepache sit in a sealed bottle in the refrigerator for an additional day to enhance carbonation.

Tips for Perfect Tepache

Use Ripe Pineapple: A ripe pineapple will yield the best flavor for tepache. It's sweeter and has more natural sugars, which helps with fermentation.

Watch the Fermentation Time: Tepache ferments quickly, especially in warm climates. Taste after 2 days to prevent over-fermentation, which can make it too sour.

Customize the Sweetness: Adjust the amount of piloncillo or brown sugar to your taste. Tepache is traditionally sweet, but you can use less sugar if you prefer a milder sweetness.

Boost Carbonation Naturally: For a slightly fizzy tepache, bottle it in a tightly sealed container and refrigerate for an additional day after straining.

Variations of Tepache

Tepache is delicious as it is, but here are a few variations you can try:

Orange Peel and Spices: Add a few pieces of orange peel and a couple of star anise pods for extra citrus and spicy notes.

Spicy Tepache: Add a small, de-seeded chile pepper to the fermentation jar for a hint of spice.

Ginger Tepache: Add a few slices of fresh ginger for a slightly spiced, refreshing flavor that pairs well with pineapple.

Mixed Fruit Tepache: Add mango peels or apple peels for additional fruity notes and a richer flavor.

Serving Suggestions

Tepache is versatile and pairs well with many meals or snacks. Here are a few ways to enjoy it:

On Ice: Serve tepache over ice with a squeeze of lime for a refreshing drink on a hot day.

As a Mixer: Tepache makes an excellent mixer for cocktails. Try it with tequila or rum for a unique, tropical twist.

With Tacos: Tepache's tangy sweetness complements spicy tacos or Mexican street food.

Frozen Tepache: Pour tepache into ice pop molds for a refreshing, frozen treat.

The Origins of Tepache

Tepache has roots in pre-Hispanic Mexico, where indigenous communities would ferment various fruits, corn, and grains for beverages. Pineapple tepache became popular over time and is now a common drink in Mexican markets and street stalls. Traditionally sold in plastic bags with straw, tepache is enjoyed by people of all ages as a natural, mildly fizzy refreshment. While commercial tepache is now available, many people continue to make it at home, using passed-down recipes that emphasize fresh ingredients and natural fermentation.

Frequently Asked Questions

Q: Can I make tepache without piloncillo?

Yes, if you don't have piloncillo, dark brown sugar is a good substitute. It provides a similar molasses-like flavor.

Q: How long does tepache last in the refrigerator?

Once strained, tepache can be stored in the refrigerator for up to a week. However, it's best enjoyed within the first few days, as it will continue to ferment slowly even in the fridge.

Q: Is tepache alcoholic?

Tepache is only mildly alcoholic, as the fermentation process is short. However, the longer it ferments, the more alcohol it can develop, so taste-test it regularly.

Q: Can I reuse the pineapple peels for a second batch?

Yes, you can reuse the peels once but add a little more sugar to help jump-start the fermentation process for the second batch.

Why You'll Love This Tepache Recipe

This tepache recipe is simple, flavorful, and a great way to enjoy homemade, refreshing Mexican flavors. With its light fizz, tangy-sweet flavor, and hint of spices, tepache is perfect for hot days or as a unique drink for gatherings. Made with just a few ingredients, it's a fun project that lets you experience traditional Mexican fermentation in your own kitchen.

Enjoy this refreshing, lightly carbonated drink with a hint of pineapple and spice—it's a delicious, natural soda that's sure to impress!

55

Tortilla Recipe

Tortillas are the foundation of countless Mexican dishes, from tacos and quesadillas to burritos and enchiladas. Corn tortillas are an ancient staple of Mexican cuisine, rooted in indigenous traditions, while flour tortillas were introduced later and are more commonly found in northern Mexico. Making tortillas from scratch is easier than you might think and delivers a fresh, authentic flavor that store-bought versions simply can't match. This chapter will guide you through making traditional corn and flour tortillas at home, complete with tips for perfecting your technique.

Corn Tortilla Recipe

Corn tortillas are made with just two ingredients: masa harina (corn flour) and water. Masa harina is a special type of corn flour that's nixtamalized, giving it a unique flavor and texture that's perfect for tortillas.

Ingredients

2 cups masa harina (such as Maseca or Bob's Red Mill)

1 1/2 cups warm water, plus extra if needed

A pinch of salt (optional)

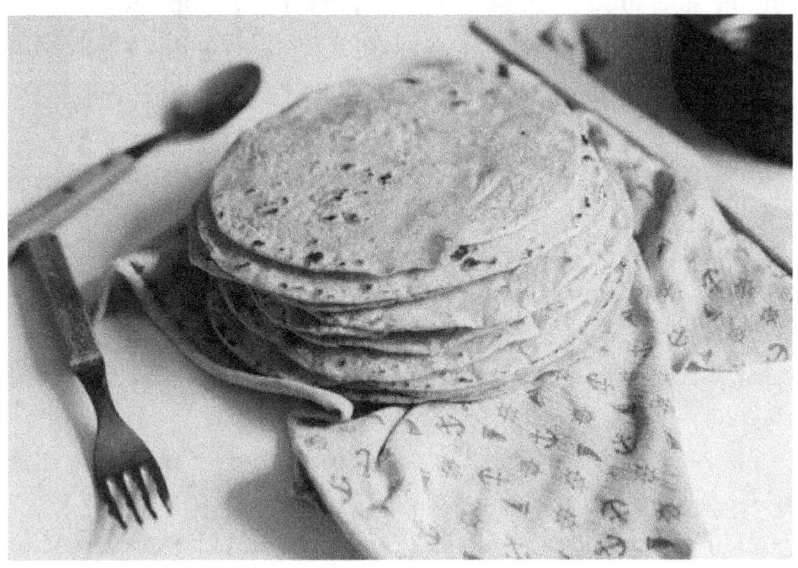

INSTRUCTIONS

Make the Dough: In a large mixing bowl, combine the masa harina with a pinch of salt, if desired. Gradually add warm water while mixing until the dough comes together. Knead the dough for about 2-3 minutes, until it's smooth and pliable. The dough should feel like soft playdough—neither too dry nor too sticky. If it's crumbly, add a bit more water; if it's too sticky, add a bit more masa harina.

Divide the Dough: Divide the dough into 12 equal portions for small tortillas (about 5-6 inches) or 8 portions for larger tortillas. Roll each portion into a ball.

Press the Tortillas: Place a ball of dough between two pieces of plastic wrap or parchment paper. Using a tortilla apress, gently press down to flatten the dough into a thin, round tortilla. If you don't have a tortilla press, use a heavy dish or a rolling pin.

Cook the Tortillas: Preheat a comal (griddle) or a large skillet over medium-high heat. Once hot, carefully peel the tortilla from the plastic and place it on the comal. Cook for about 30-40 seconds on one side, until small brown spots appear, then flip and cook for another 30 seconds. Flip once more to let it puff slightly, which gives the tortilla a fluffy texture. Adjust cooking time based on thickness and heat level.

Keep Warm: Place cooked tortillas in a clean kitchen towel or tortilla warmer to keep them warm and soft. Serve immediately or reheat them briefly on the comal when ready to use.

Tips for Perfect Corn Tortillas

Adjust the Water: Masa harina brands vary slightly, so you may need to adjust the water. Add it gradually and adjust as needed until the dough feels smooth.

Press Evenly: Press tortillas evenly for consistent thickness; they should be thin but not see-through.

Flip Carefully: Corn tortillas can be fragile. Use a spatula to flip them gently, especially if the dough is on the moist side.

Flour Tortilla Recipe

Flour tortillas, known for their soft, pliable texture, are typically used in northern Mexican cuisine. They're made with wheat flour and are great for burritos, quesadillas, and wraps. This recipe includes lard or butter for richness, but you can substitute vegetable oil if you prefer.

Ingredients

2 cups of all-purpose flour

1/2 tsp baking powder

1/2 tsp salt

3 tbsp lard, butter, or vegetable oil

3/4 cup warm water

Instructions

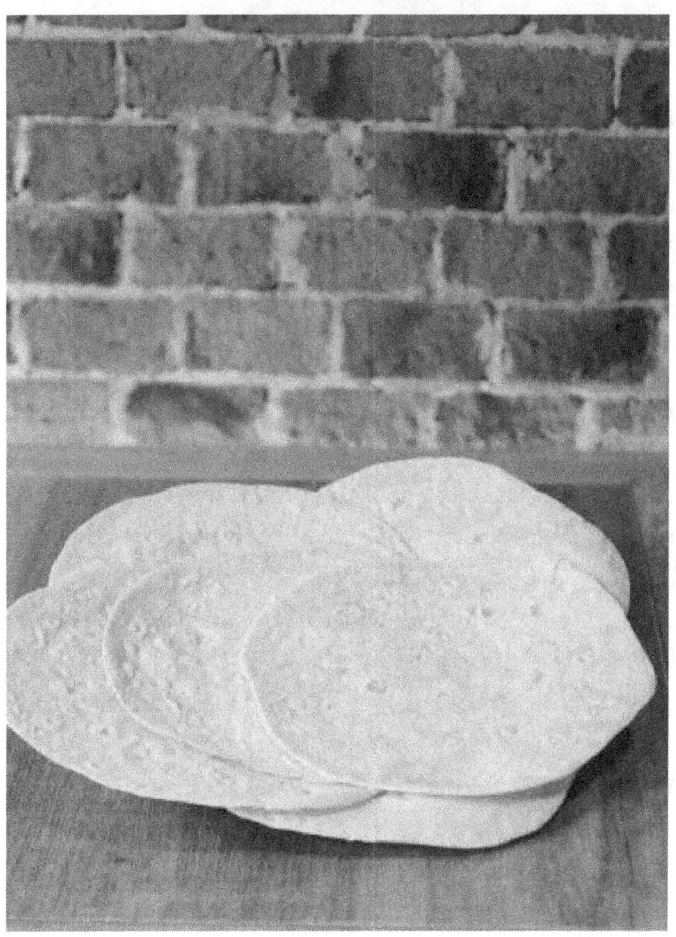

COMBINE DRY INGREDIENTS: In a large bowl, whisk together the flour, baking powder, and salt.

Add Fat: Add the lard, butter, or oil to the dry ingredients. Use your fingers or a pastry cutter to mix until the mixture resembles coarse crumbs.

Add Water and Knead: Gradually add the warm water, mix until the dough comes together. Knead the dough for 5-7 minutes, until smooth and elastic. The dough should be soft but not sticky.

Rest the Dough: Cover the dough with a kitchen towel or plastic wrap and let it rest for at least 15-30 minutes. Resting allows the gluten to relax, making the tortillas easier to roll out.

Divide and Roll Out: Divide the dough into 8-12 equal portions, depending on the size of tortillas you want. Roll each portion into a ball. On a lightly floured surface, use a rolling pin to roll each ball into a thin circle, about 8-10 inches in diameter.

Cook the Tortillas: Heat a comal or skillet over medium-high heat. Place a rolled tortilla on the hot comal and cook for about 30 seconds to 1 minute, until you see bubbles forming. Flip and cook for another 30 seconds, or until light brown spots appear.

Keep Warm: Stack the cooked tortillas in a clean kitchen towel or tortilla warmer to keep them soft. Serve warm or reheat as needed.

Tips for Perfect Flour Tortillas

Don't Skip the Rest: Allowing the dough to rest makes it easier to roll out and results in softer tortillas.

Use Just Enough Flour for Rolling: Use minimal flour for rolling, as too much can make tortillas dry.

Adjust Heat as Needed: If the tortillas are browning too quickly, lower the heat to ensure they cook evenly.

Storing and Reheating Tortillas

Corn Tortillas: Store leftover corn tortillas in a sealed plastic bag in the refrigerator for up to 5 days. Reheat on a hot comal or skillet to restore softness.

Flour Tortillas: Store leftover flour tortillas in an airtight container or zip-top bag at room temperature for up to 3 days or refrigerate for up to a week. Reheat on a skillet or in the microwave, covered with a damp paper towel.

Serving Suggestions for Tortillas

Corn Tortillas: Use for tacos, enchiladas, tostadas, and quesadillas. Corn tortillas are also ideal for chilaquiles and can be cut into chips for salsas and dips.

Flour Tortillas: Use for burritos, quesadillas, fajitas, wraps, and as a soft base for taco fillings. They're great for breakfast burritos and can also be cut and fried for tortilla chips.

Frequently Asked Questions

Q: Can I make corn tortillas without a tortilla press?

Yes! A rolling pin works just fine. Place the masa between plastic wrap or parchment paper, then roll out gently until thin.

Q: Can I substitute oil for lard in flour tortillas?

Yes, vegetable oil or butter can be used in place of lard. Lard provides the most authentic flavor, but other fats will still yield delicious tortillas.

Q: What's the difference between corn and flour tortillas?

Corn tortillas have a more rustic, earthy flavor and are naturally gluten-free. Flour tortillas are softer, more flexible, and often used for larger, rolled dishes like burritos.

Q: How do I keep tortillas soft?

Store tortillas in a warm, moist environment, like a covered tortilla warmer or a towel. Keeping them covered helps maintain softness and flexibility. Making corn and flour tortillas from scratch is a rewarding way to bring authentic Mexican flavors into your home. Corn tortillas offer a taste of tradition and pair beautifully with Mexican classics, while flour tortillas add a soft, pillowy base for hearty fillings. With a few basic ingredients and some practice, you'll be able to make fresh, delicious tortillas that elevate any Mexican meal. Whether you're crafting tacos, burritos, or enchiladas, these homemade tortillas are sure to add a genuine touch to your dishes.

www.ingramcontent.com/pod-product-compliance
Lightning Source LLC
Chambersburg PA
CBHW071356150726
48000CB00001B/40